Restless Legs Syndrome

The RLS Rebel's Survival Guide

D1545803

Jill Gunzel

aka The RLS Rebel

Restless Legs Syndrome: The RLS Rebel's Survival Guide

Published by Wheatmark™
610 East Delano Street, Suite 104, Tucson, Arizona 85705 U.S.A.
www.wheatmark.com

International Standard Book Number: 1-58736-579-0
Library of Congress Control Number: 2006920415

Photos by Arizona Photo Solutions
http://www.azphotosolutions.com
Front cover: *The RLS Rebel choking the RLS Bully* (see Preface)

To RLSers: Past, Present, and Future.

To my father and grandmother,
who knew the feeling of
"a hollow leg" and "ants crawling under the skin,"
but not the name "RLS."

To current RLS rebels
who are tenaciously fighting back.

To my grandchildren and all future RLSers,
who will hopefully be blessed with a cure.

ACKNOWLEDGEMENTS

MY ENDLESS APPRECIATION goes to my husband, Steve. He stuck with me through our teenage dates, while I squirmed and complained. Later, he understood when I had to walk the floors rather than cuddle with him in bed. He listened faithfully to new ideas and chapter revisions, while joking that he knew the back of my head better than my face. (Too many days at the computer will cause that to happen.) When chemotherapy made me bald, he lovingly rubbed my head and encouraged me to keep writing.

Special thanks go to my mother, Alma Vactor, who patiently massaged my legs when I was young. Though she didn't know why her husband and daughter couldn't be still, she was always there to comfort us. She patiently listened to me practice my RLS Rebel Program presentations and never complained when I used her living room to create Arl and other rebel program props. Her encouragement was endless.

I thank my children for attending my presentations and encouraging my efforts. My daughter, Julie Graff, was the first to show me the humor in RLS, when she renamed it "Ridiculous Legs Syndrome." I wish to thank her husband, Jeremy Graff, for his attempts to help with my manuscript, despite my stubbornness. And thanks to their daughter, Leslie, who exhibited what appeared to be classic RLS symptoms during her first year of life. She gave me added incentive to finish this book and pass along what I have learned.

Thanks go to my son and his wife, Jon and Trina Gunzel (Arizona Photo Solutions), for the great job they did on the cover photos and their encouragement to share the RLS Rebel Program on a larger scale. I can't tell if their two-year-old son, Wyatt, has RLS wiggles or just loves clogging as much as I do. If he has RLS, his love of dancing will be the first trick in his Bag of Tricks.

Special thanks to my friend and fellow clogging instructor, Chriss Burhmester. Though he has never had RLS, Chriss learned about it in detail after going over every word of my manuscript with the same pickiness we apply to our clogging cue sheets. I especially thank him for sticking with me through days when I was too sick from chemotherapy to think straight. He knew just when to push and gently encouraged me to finish the manuscript, get well, and get back on the dance floor.

To the many friends who understood when I couldn't "play" because I had to finish this book, I thank you, and I'm warning you, "I'm back!" It's time to go shopping, talk on the phone for hours, clog to our hearts' content, and celebrate life. Thank you for waiting for me.

I am grateful to over 1,000 RLSers from the Yahoo.com email support group "rlssupport." Many of them started as cyberfriends, but became true "real time" friends through the years. I thank those who fought with me about my ideas; their criticisms and objections helped me formulate a program that applies to all RLSers. I never could have survived some of those heated debates if it weren't for other group members who kept me focused and encouraged me to stay positive and keep sharing my ideas. I am thankful for your encouragement and friendship.

I appreciate the numerous healthcare providers who have asked to share my program with other RLSers. Dr. Henig, thank you for always keeping me accurate with my comments and for asking me to contribute to your book.

Dr. Buchfuhrer, thank you for sharing authorship of a chapter with me and for asking to reference my book in yours. Both of you gave me a sense of credibility that helped me believe in this book. I am grateful to Dr. Patrick Hogan and Sharon Jung, from the Tacoma Area RLS Support Group. Your feedback and desire to give copies of my manual to your patients helped me see the importance of making the RLS Rebel Program readily available to RLSers and health-care providers.

I wish to thank Drs. Richard Allen, Wayne Henig, David Rye, Bruce Ehrenberg, and Charles Adler for graciously sharing the stage with a lay RLSer, and for treating the RLS Rebel Program and myself with continued professional respect. I was always proud to join with you in presenting a program that balanced pertinent medical information about RLS with valuable self-help information for RLSers.

I thank Dr. Arthur Walters for his enthusiastic response to my presentation at the 2004 RLS Foundation national conference and for his positive response to the RLS Rebel Program manual. I have been honored beyond imagination by the exceptional quote he provided for the back cover of this book.

Special inspiration came from invitations to present my program to support groups in San Antonio, Tacoma, Portland, and Tucson. My thanks go to Barbara Acosta, Newt Hagar, Marian Cooter, and the Tucson support group leader for helping me see the importance of sharing the RLS Rebel Program.

And finally, having saved one of the best for last, I thank the RLS Foundation for recognizing the value of the RLS Rebel Program and allowing me to be a part of their efforts to educate the world about RLS. Through their continued efforts to promote research and coordinate RLS information, thousands are supported and hope for a cure is kept alive.

CONTENTS

RLS Rebel Program
PART II: THE BAG OF TRICKS APPROACH (BOTA)

Understanding the BOTA
No easy route. It's an approach. Four steps of the BOTA. The BOTA file system.

Step 1: Gather Your Tricks
Why not one trick? Two types of tricks. Three warnings about tricks. Keep detailed records.

Step 2: Pack Your Bags
Pack selectively. Plan ahead. Pack combinations of no-prop and prop tricks. Pack different tricks for different types of RLS. Keep a packing list for each activity. Lighten and adjust your BOT. Review, repack, and restock.

Step 3: Plan of Attack
What if RLS symptoms show up? A whole new concept. Develop a two-stage Plan of Attack. The *preparation stage.* The *attack stage.* Ammunition for your attack stage. Start your attack early. Don't let RLS disable you.

Step 4: Relief Plans
Understand the difference in Plan of Attack and Relief Plan. Do Relief Plans always require you to stop the activity? Practice *zero tolerance.* Alternate between Step 3 and Step 4. Develop several Relief Plans. Is the BOTA a ridiculous waste of time? Not-so-popular Relief Plans. Focus on successes.

YOUR BAG OF TRICKS

Does this mean I always have to carry a BOT? Consider variety, purpose, and timing. Your BOT contents will constantly change. Keep your BOT handy.

Use *zero tolerance*. Think of walking as a blessing. Simulate walking. Stretching exercises. Use massage and brushing. Practice the skillful art of *bully noise*. Take fast deep breaths. Consider sex. Distraction.

Prepare your mind. Carefully choose your focus. Discipline yourself to stay focused. Believe it will work. Consider these tips.

No-prop or prop? Consider direct input. Consider portability. Carefully choose headphones. Try a sound pillow or pillow speaker. Explore other audio options. Listen analytically and intently. Don't resist. Record your techniques.

Potential disadvantages of prop tricks. Choosing your prop tricks. Alternative medical systems. Biologically-based treatments. Manipulative and body-based methods. Mind-body interventions. Energy therapies. The *bar of soap trick*: Effective prop or placebo? Keep searching.

Start your research. Keep good notes. Reasons to postpone pharmaceutical use. Rebellious thoughts about pharmaceuticals. Drugs are *wimping out* or drugs are *assisted living*. Drugs are a *last resort* or drugs can be early intervention. Drugs make you dependent or drugs keep you independent. Drugs cure RLS or drugs relieve RLS symptoms. The doctor dictates drug use or the patient communicates needs. Use a drug approved for RLS or use the best medications for current needs. Rely on drugs or rely on a diverse BOT with pharmaceuticals and alternatives. Four categories of drug options. Prescription and intravenous iron treatments. Don't let your prescription drugs deplete you. Keep the big picture in mind.

When in doubt, ask questions. Be a little skeptical, but don't lose hope.

MORE REBEL ATTITUDES and AMMUNITION

Be a parental rebel. Start your child's RLS Rebel Program file system. RLS and babies. Treat with sleep. Convey positive outlooks and feelings of empowerment. Listen carefully to descriptions of symptoms. Teach *zero tolerance*. Emphasize no-prop tricks. Talk with teachers. Teach responsibility and politeness. Teach children about *bully noise* and mental distraction tricks. Teach children to pack and use their BOT. Prethink your responses. Convey happiness and support.

The RLS Rebel's Survival Guide. Your RLS rebel patient. RLS Rebel Program tips. Teamwork creates the ultimate in complementary medicine.

The vicious cycle of RLS and sleep deprivation. Learn more about sleep and sleep deprivation. Consider how daytime activities affect your sleep. Do foods or supplements affect your sleep? Be aware of your thoughts about getting to sleep. Develop your wind-down routine. Use sleep-inducing words and images. Middle-of-the-night wake ups. Common middle-of-the-night mistakes. Try some unpleasant Relief Plans. You and your sleep partner. The *snuggle trick.*

BOTA Step 1: Gather Your Tricks (for all RLS situations). BOTA Step 2: Pack Your Bags (for getting to sleep). BOTA Step 3: Plan of Attack (for getting to sleep). BOTA Step 4: Relief Plans (for stopping symptoms).

Hospitalizations. Disasters and accidents. Kidney disease and dialysis. Chemotherapy. Pregnancy. When an RLSer is bed-ridden. Work situations. Theaters/movies/concerts. Stroke and paralysis. Exhaustion and personal safety.

Stowing your travel BOT. Pack your travel BOT. Plan of Attack: *Preparation stage.* Plan of Attack: *Attack stage.* Relief Plans for air travel. Pay attention to the return trip.

Prepare for the role of RLS rebel supporter. The many hats you wear. Use the RLS Rebel Program. Sometimes you have to take charge. Socialization and emotional health. Supporting children who have RLS. Relationships. Appearances can be deceiving. Just be a friend.

Help find the cure. Become a more skillful RLS rebel. Be still! RLS affirmations and reminders. Best wishes for restful moments and peaceful nights.

PREFACE

I HAVE DEALT WITH RLS symptoms since I was six years old. My father must have had RLS, too, because he often walked the floors at night, complaining of a "hollow leg feeling."

My mother used to say, "Your father flies his airplane in his sleep," (probably a sign of Periodic Limb Movement Disorder).

My grandmother complained of feeling as if ants were crawling under her skin, and she spent many nights soaking in a hot bath. My mother began complaining of RLS symptoms after her stroke in 1999. My brother has RLS. My uncle has RLS. My two children have it. One grandbaby acts like she has it. A cousin in Australia has it, and was shocked when I noticed and identified his typical RLS squirm while we drove home from seeing the Grand Canyon.

When I think of all the people who have had to struggle with this awful syndrome, it makes me want to choke the *RLS bully*. My expression in the cover photo aptly represents my frustration as I'm trying to choke Arl (a visual aid used during my talks about RLS). The nickname *Arl* came from the sound of the R-L in RLS. Arl is an ugly mask sitting on an IV pole that telescopes to seven feet high, representing the out-of-control *beast of RLS*. After I explain the RLS Rebel Program's Reduction Plan, Arl retracts to five feet high, representing the obnoxious, but controllable *RLS bully* (complete with a propeller-topped beanie).

In lieu of being able to choke RLS out of my life, I developed the RLS Rebel Program. Arl and I have presented this program at six regional meetings and one national conference of the RLS Foundation and to RLS support groups in four states. The positive feedback from RLSers and the kudos I received from many RLS medical professionals have made me realize the need to reach more RLSers. They needed something they could hold and use as a reference. It was time to make the program available in a book. I hope you will get a chance to see Arl in action, but until then, this book will help you develop your own guide to surviving with RLS.

The chapters of the first section, "Introductions," give a brief description of RLS, the differences in RLS and Periodic Limb Movement Disorder (PLMD), RLS rebel terminology, and the general points of the RLS Rebel Program. You will also find quick-start tips for managing your RLS, and a chapter of frequently asked questions.

The RLS Rebel Program has two parts: the Reduction Plan and the BOTA (Bag of Tricks Approach). The six steps of the Reduction Plan are described in the second section of this book, "The RLS Rebel Program: Part I–The Reduction Plan." By following these steps, you will learn to reduce the frequency and severity of your RLS symptoms.

The third section, "The RLS Rebel Program: Part II–The BOTA," explains the four steps of the Bag of Tricks Approach. By following these steps, you will learn to manage all your RLS treatment options. You will learn to prepare for at-rest activities with a combination of tricks and to apply those tricks in a well-developed approach.

The fourth section, "Your Bag of Tricks," describes two main groups of treatment options: prop tricks and no-prop tricks. Various chapters detail the important tricks of using prescription drugs, concentration, and music. A final chapter of the section gives tips for deciding whether a treatment is worth trying.

The fifth section, "More Rebel Attitudes and Ammunition," offers additional survival tactics, including chapters on how to help children who have RLS, how to develop teamwork with your RLS healthcare providers, sleep tips, RLS travel advice, and how to manage other special RLS-provoking situations.

Restless Legs Syndrome: The RLS Rebel's Survival Guide will not reveal a cure for RLS. Instead, this book will show you how to become rebellious, fight back, and take control over your life before Arl makes a total mess of it. You will learn how to develop a file system and how to track all the unique variables and details affecting your own RLS survival. I encourage you to learn the RLS Rebel Program and become an RLS rebel.

There are no easy answers to surviving with RLS. When I give talks about the RLS Rebel Program, I usually wear a pair of overalls. I tell my audience the overalls are a visual aid, meant to remind them of the hard work and commitment it takes to survive with RLS. As you read this book, put on your own virtual pair of overalls and prepare to work hard. With determination and a good rebellious attitude, you will soon benefit from your labor.

Jill Gunzel,
aka The RLS Rebel

INTRODUCTIONS

The RLS Rebel

Disclaimer: This survival guide is a resource of ideas developed by someone who has Restless Legs Syndrome. I claim no professional medical background. I do not intend anything to be medical advice or a substitute for what your doctor prescribes or recommends. And I do not claim or imply that my ideas are a cure or that they will work for everyone.

Who is the RLS Rebel?

I REMEMBER FEELING AN irresistible urge to wiggle when I was six years old. As a teenager, I was told it was *growing pains*. My inability to sit still became a problem in school, on dates, and when traveling. In my twenties, the irresistible urge began affecting my arms. In my thirties, it often prevented my ability to get to sleep. In my forties, the attacks lasted all night and left my limbs in pain the next day. At that point, I felt sleep deprived, panicked, and victimized. Besides referring to it as *my leg thing*, I avoided mentioning it to people, lest they think I was crazy.

In January 1998, I searched the Internet and found the Restless Legs Syndrome Foundation. That is when I learned *my leg thing* was called Restless Legs Syndrome (RLS). I immediately joined a wonderful email support group and began analyzing my RLS experience and searching for more effective responses. After years of being a victim, I felt a sense of rebellion and decided to fight back.

As I discovered more information about RLS and how to fight back, I wanted to share what I had learned, with others. I created a website where I could detail what I knew and encourage others to take up their own fight against RLS. Determined to keep RLS from destroying my life and wanting to empower other RLSers (people experiencing RLS) to adopt rebellious attitudes, I began referring to myself as the RLS Rebel. In April 2000, at the first national meeting of the RLS Foundation, I distributed a handout titled "Attitudes of an RLS Rebel." The material from this handout can be seen in the "Quick Start Tips" chapter of this book.

I knew I could not offer a cure, but I was sure I could encourage people to do a better job of surviving with RLS. At first, I spoke and wrote about alternative treatments and self-help approaches to dealing with RLS. Later, in preparation for a speech at the March 2001 regional conference of the RLS Foundation, I developed a comprehensive approach that included the option of using prescription medications. I called my approach "The RLS Rebel Program." It was based on a two-part outline RLSers could follow to guide their fight against RLS.

In September 2001, I began distributing my manual, *The RLS Rebel Program: A Survival Guide for People with Restless Legs Syndrome*. During the next three years, I received valuable feedback from people who had heard me speak about the RLS Rebel Program or had read my manual. That feedback led to many revisions and additions to the manual. In November 2004, I decided to make the information available as the book you are now reading. This guide is based on my RLS website and manual, but also contains a great deal of new information.

The information in this guide has helped me reduce the severity and frequency of my RLS symptoms and has helped me respond effectively to any remaining RLS attacks. I have found ways to continue many activities that previously had been difficult—and sometimes impossible—to enjoy. My most exciting progress has been learning to get to sleep, even during an RLS attack. I refuse to be frightened by theories that RLS gets worse with age. Instead of worrying about whether it will get worse, I focus on improving my ability to respond quickly and successfully to RLS attacks. I suspect that more things will aggravate my RLS as I age, but with skillful application of the information in this book, I can reduce the severity and frequency of my attacks and greatly improve my ability to control my RLS. At this rate, my experience with RLS should improve, not worsen, as I get older.

Close to 50 years of personal experience with RLS has made me eager to rebel, gain control, and share my findings and successes with others. My master's degree in education and my bachelor's degree in public speaking have helped me bring the information to others through conferences, the Internet, and workshops. I hope this book will encourage RLSers to take charge and feel empowered to win their battles against RLS.

Who else can be an RLS rebel?

A rebel is a person who rises against authority or oppression and possesses a great deal of independence in thought and action. Anyone who has lived with RLS has felt the oppression and restrictiveness of its presence. If you have decided you hate the feeling of being victimized by RLS and have decided to fight back, then you have already become an RLS rebel. Being an RLS rebel is much more than just wishing for a miraculous cure. It is a decision to fight back by investing a great deal of time and effort into developing reliable survival strategies.

To be an RLS rebel is to recognize the complexity and slippery nature of this disorder. RLS rebels have to be ready to collect information, plan for RLS attacks, prepare appropriate responses, and quickly change plans when everything suddenly acts or responds differently than expected. Alertness and eagerness to continue learning are all necessary qualities of an RLS rebel.

Friends, family, supporters, and caregivers can be RLS rebels, too. If you want your loved ones to support you more effectively or if you are someone who is supporting an RLSer, be sure to read the chapter "To Those Who Support Us."

Many medical professionals are RLS rebels, eager to provide effective treatments and relief for their patients. Both the patient and doctor can use this survival guide as the framework for their teamed efforts to conduct an offensive against RLS. Medical professionals should pay particular attention to the chapters "To Our RLS Healthcare Providers" and "Do's and Don'ts for Dealing with Your Doctor."

An RLS rebel recognizes there is no easy fix or cure for RLS. If you are an RLS rebel, you have made a commitment to invest a good deal of effort into successfully managing RLS in your own life, in the life of a patient or client, or in the life of a friend or loved one. I congratulate you on your decision to take charge and fight back.

RLS Basics

Are you sure you have RLS?

THIS IS A trick question. We do not have a sure-fire test for Restless Legs Syndrome (RLS). Instead, we have to ask whether our complaints match the commonly used criteria for diagnosing RLS. If you have RLS, you will probably answer yes to the following questions:

1. **Do you experience irresistible urges to move your limbs?** The urges lead you to voluntarily move your limbs, as opposed to making your limbs jerk without your say-so. Of course, you do not feel you have a choice but to move.

2. **Do the urges to wiggle tend to happen more when you attempt at-rest activities?** Symptoms are likely to hit while you are watching TV, at the movies, at a concert, reading, riding in a car or airplane, or trying to be still in bed.

3. **Do the urges stop when you walk, stretch, or become mentally distracted?** Movement and mental distraction are reliable methods for stopping the urges. The urges may return as soon as you resume your at-rest activity.

4. **Do the urges tend to occur more in the late afternoon or evening?** Most people's first RLS experiences begin in the late afternoon or evening. Around 4:00 a.m., many people find their symptoms are relieved. In some cases,

however, symptoms can start in the morning and occur any time of day.

Other symptoms, such as pain, exhaustion, insomnia, burning sensations, and tingling can be associated with RLS, but the four criteria (listed above) need to happen in order to be confident you are dealing with RLS.

What causes RLS?

There are numerous theories about what causes RLS. Many believe it is a disorder of the central nervous system, but to date, no definitive cause has been found. Some studies suggest RLS may be related to amounts of iron in the brain, while other studies show a relationship to dopamine. Even when we think we have discovered something to be true about RLS (e.g., its probable cause, its behavior, its response to treatments), we inevitably discover the information is not true for all RLSers.

It appears there are two types of RLS. *Primary RLS* is probably inherited, is experienced by others in the family, and is usually present during childhood years. *Secondary RLS* usually occurs later in life and has an onset that may be attributable to a coexisting medical condition or treatment (e.g., surgery, back injury, diabetes, peripheral neuropathy, prescription medications, pregnancy). The occurrence of primary RLS in multiple family members leads us to believe there is a genetic link. The sudden onset of secondary RLS suggests a trauma or sudden change in the body, resulting in irresistible urges to move.

I have a theory about what causes RLS. My theory might be totally wrong, but for now, it helps me formulate my strategies for taking control over my RLS survival. I believe RLS is caused by one or more occurrences that stress us mentally, physically, emotionally, or spiritually. When our systems become stressed, I believe it sends us into an instinctual fight-

or-flight response. Subconsciously, we feel unsettled, out of balance, or unsafe, and our body and mind tell us we need to flee, move, wiggle, or run to safety. We may have a chemical imbalance, a physical injury, stress from another ailment, or a major change in our lifestyle, diet, or nutritional needs. Any of these situations could change our natural balance, cause us to be unsettled, and create an urge to move.

Will it get worse?

The big question on the mind of many RLSers is: Will it get worse as we get older? If they have already tried several prescription medications and alternative treatments, they may panic at the thought of possibly running out of options if their symptoms get worse. Much of the literature about RLS says it *tends* to get worse with age.

Though it is common to have more RLS symptoms as we get older, I am not convinced it is due to one specific thing degenerating and causing the increased symptoms. As we age, we all deal with more imbalances and more stresses to our systems. I believe it is the added aggravation of those additional imbalances and stresses that leads to new RLS symptoms and an increase in the severity of symptoms we already experience.

Studies have shown less iron in brain cells from people who had RLS than in cells from those who did not have RLS. Despite lower levels of iron in the brain cells, there is no evidence of those iron-deficient cells being damaged. These findings and the lack of proof that something has degenerated or been permanently damaged, lead me to believe RLS is not caused by something that gets worse with age.

For those who relate well to analogies, try this one. If you led a relatively inactive life, your wardrobe may last many years. You would not need anything special and you would not be putting a great deal of stress on the clothes in your closet. Your wardrobe would continue working for you as long as you and your lifestyle did not change. However, if your weight changed, you became more active, or you started a variety of new adventures (e.g., swimming, biking, traveling, hunting, square dancing), you might find your wardrobe severely lacking or inappropriate. Did the wardrobe change? Did it suddenly become a closet of changed or damaged clothing? No. Your lifestyle and your requirements changed, resulting in a problematic wardrobe.

I believe our RLS (like the clothes in the closet) does not get worse just because we get older. I believe it is the changes in our lives, imbalances in our systems, deficiencies, and new aggravators, which increase the severity and frequency of our RLS.

The important thing to realize is that we can often change the variables affecting our symptoms. We can avoid many RLS-provoking at-rest activities (e.g., not go to a movie, not read a book), until we have better treatments for our symptoms. In many cases, rather than avoiding situations, we can treat for them and overcome the symptoms with effective therapies and responses. This ability to adjust variables and treat symptoms means we need not worry about RLS getting worse with age.

Control is the real issue

Though we all question how severe our RLS is and whether it will get worse, the important question is: Do you feel as if you are able to control your experience with RLS? Can you prevent symptoms? Can you avoid situations where RLS is likely to occur? Are you able to respond effectively to stop RLS symptoms? Many RLSers think they have severe symptoms when they actually have mild symptoms, but have no way to control their experience with those symptoms. Once they develop some effective responses and learn how to reduce aggravating factors, their control enables them to proceed with relative ease.

Many RLSers manage their at-rest activities quite well, despite their severe RLS symptoms. With proper treatments and careful planning, even the most severe cases of RLS can be brought under control and the RLSer can feel empowered, rather than victimized. A person with severe RLS will have to invest much more effort in controlling symptoms and managing at-rest activities, but the investment will be well worth the time.

To insure your ability to have control over your RLS, even if symptoms get worse as you get older, it is important to begin developing your rebellious habits. Learn to fight back. Someday, you may have a severe case of RLS and need more abilities and more control. If you start early, you will be ready for anything. I always say, "I don't care if the RLS gets worse, as long as I keep getting better at responding to it." It must just be my rebel attitude.

You can have control of your RLS and still experience severe symptoms. As I started controlling my severe RLS symptoms, other RLSers told me, "You probably never really had RLS." After I explained how I was able to get to sleep, despite an ongoing RLS attack, another RLSer told me, "Your symptoms probably weren't that bad. I could never do that. Just wait. Yours will get worse."

The ability to control your symptoms with the systematic and skillful application of treatments doesn't mean you do not have severe RLS. You can be in control, or not in control, whether your symptoms are mild or severe. Your RLS survival is a reflection of how well you apply your survival program, regardless of the severity of your RLS.

Is it mild, moderate, or severe RLS?

We do not have a reliable way to rate the severity of someone's RLS. Some scales rate RLS according to intensity of symptoms. Some rate it according to frequency or time of day when symptoms occur. Others note whether symptoms are just in the legs, or whether they also occur in the arms, trunk, or face. In 2004, the Restless Legs Syndrome Foundation's medical advisory board published an algorithm for the management of RLS. This formula for solving the RLS treatment dilemma describes treatments for three categories of RLS: intermittent, daily, and refractory (meaning the RLS did not respond well to previous treatment with a dopamine agonist). The algorithm provides a valuable tool for medical professionals treating RLS patients, but still does not provide an accurate method to rate the severity of every person's experience with RLS.

The most common tendency is to rate RLS severity according to what treatments are used. If you use only alternative (self-help) methods, it is usually assumed you have mild RLS. If you use mostly alternative methods but need to use prescription medications some of the time, it is usually assumed you have moderate RLS. If you use only prescription medications because self-help methods seem ineffective, it is usually assumed you have severe RLS. There are many problems with this thinking.

1. Prescription medicines can be useful in mild RLS situations, and need not be restricted to out-of-control severe cases. Therefore, it is incorrect to say that use of prescription medicine is an indicator of RLS severity.

2. Some cases of severe RLS are controlled without use of prescription medications. Therefore, it is incorrect to say the absence of prescription medication use is an indicator of mild RLS.

If the type of treatment is not the determining factor in rating the severity of one's RLS, what is?

The RLS Rebel's rating system:
Frequency, type, and effort

When I rate a person's RLS, I look at several factors. Though a single factor may be present to an extreme (making the RLS seem severe), RLS severity should be rated according to the combination of factors. If they are all at the extreme or intense end of the scale, the RLS is severe. If some factors are intense but others are mild or infrequent, the person has moderate RLS, and if the RLSer reports only slight occurrence of all these factors, the RLS is probably mild.

1. **Frequency:** Mild cases of RLS tend to begin late in the day, during the evening, or during the night. Symptoms may occur intermittently, providing many nights with no symptoms. As the RLS becomes more severe, the person might begin to have daily RLS. These symptoms might also begin appearing earlier in the day. If symptoms appear first thing in the morning and occur on a daily basis, we might say the high *frequency* would indicate a potentially severe case of RLS.

2. **Type:** Mild cases of RLS tend to occur in the legs, and consist of irresistible urges to move. Moderate and severe cases of RLS might involve arms, trunk, or face. These more intense cases might also involve muscle tightening and pain. The more intense types of RLS, involving more parts of the body and more physical reactions, including pain, are indications of potentially severe RLS.

3. **Effort:** Mild cases of RLS might be relieved by standing up for a moment or just shifting positions. Moderate cases will need more of a response. Severe cases will require carefully planned responses, including practiced skills or use of assistive devices (e.g., medications, massages, herbal remedies). The more severe the RLS, the

more effort the RLSer must put into stopping and pre-venting the attacks.

In my rating system, all three factors must be in the severe range in order to call a person's RLS *severe*. We might see a scenario where a person's symptoms start early in the morning and occur daily (a severe range for *frequency*), but the symptoms create only a slight irritation in the legs (a mild range for *type*), and are quickly relieved by a shift of position or a short walk (a mild range for *effort*). With only one factor in the severe range, I would say this person had a mild to moderate case of RLS.

In another situation, we might see someone whose RLS occurs daily (a severe range for *frequency*), involves legs and arms, is accompanied by pain (a severe range for *type*), and requires a combination of medications and self-help therapies that must be constantly and expertly used (a severe range for *effort*). This person would be experiencing a severe case of RLS.

If a person had two out of the three factors in the severe range, they might be said to have a moderate case of RLS. For instance, the person may not have symptoms daily (a mild range for *frequency*), but symptoms are painful and involve the arms (a severe range for *type*), and it takes constant effort to prevent or respond to symptoms (a severe range for *effort*).

All three levels of RLS can occur with or without the RLSer's ability to remain in control and manage the symptoms. A person could have a mild, but out-of-control case. By the same token, a person could have a severe case and be well in control, using a very effective management plan.

If I were to rate my own RLS, I would begin by rating it according to how it would be if I put no effort into managing it. I would have symptoms early in the day and on a daily basis (a severe range of *frequency*). Symptoms would occur in my legs, arms, or face, and often involve muscle tightening (a severe range for *type*), and I would need to put a great deal of effort into preventing and responding to symptoms (a severe range for *effort*). I figure my RLS is severe, but my control has improved drastically over the years, making my RLS seem mild to moderate. I went from being totally out of control, losing sleep, and giving up at-rest activities to being able to enjoy many of those activities and get a good quantity of sleep on a regular basis. Quality of sleep, however, is a different issue for another book.

Rebel Terminology

THE FOLLOWING UNIQUE terms and concepts are used throughout this book. They are words and terminology I have coined specifically for discussing my rebellious approach to Restless Legs Syndrome (RLS). More thorough explanations and definitions will be found in the following chapters.

RLSer: This term refers to anyone who experiences RLS symptoms. It avoids the need to use terms with negative implications (e.g., RLS victim, RLS sufferer).

The RLS REBEL: This is the nickname I took for myself. Now, I use "the RLS Rebel" to refer to myself, but I use "an RLS rebel" to refer to anyone who rebels against RLS, recognizes the absence of an easy fix, and commits to the hard work of applying the RLS Rebel Program.

TRICKS: I use the term *tricks* when referring to RLS treatment options because all RLS therapies remind me of magic tricks. Sometimes they work and sometimes they don't. When they do work, they often give the illusion of having cured our RLS, when they have only brought us temporary relief.

The RLS REBEL PROGRAM: This is a two-part program, readily adaptable to a file or notebook organizing system. It is used to organize your strategies for fighting back against RLS. Part I is the Reduction Plan. Part II is the Bag of Tricks Approach (BOTA).

The BEAST OF RLS: This is not a term I coined, but one that is used by many RLSers. When RLSers feel totally victimized by out-of-control RLS symptoms, it is common to hear them refer to their RLS as the *beast of RLS*.

The REDUCTION PLAN: This is the first half of the RLS Rebel Program Outline. The six steps of the Reduction Plan are based on the theory we can reduce the out-of-control *beast of RLS* and bring him down to bully size by adjusting certain variables.

The RLS BULLY: With careful and continuous application of the RLS Rebel Program Outline, the *beast of RLS* can be reduced to bully size. The *RLS bully* is still obnoxious and troublesome, but RLSers can feel powerful against the *RLS bully* and fight back effectively.

The BOT and BOTA: These letters stand for *Bag of Tricks* and *Bag of Tricks Approach*. The BOTA consists of four steps. The first two steps (the BOT) deal with gathering and assigning potentially useful tricks. The third and fourth steps (the A) deal with the approach or methods for applying and using the tricks.

ZERO TOLERANCE: This is an attitude of intolerance, leading RLSers to manage symptoms quickly. The longer an RLS attack continues, the harder it is to stop. Apply *zero tolerance*, even if all you do is get up and walk.

BULLY NOISE: RLS attacks occur when the mind and body are at-rest. Creating an active (noisy) mind can be a useful RLS trick. Similar to the practice of using white noise, *bully noise* drowns out one noise with another. It is based on old playground lessons that taught us we could block out the sounds of a bully by sticking our fingers in our ears and yelling louder than him. If RLSers can view RLS symptoms as the *bully* and find ways to keep their brain activity busier than the bully's silly taunts to wiggle, they can actually overpower the urge to move.

Frequently Asked Survival Questions

1. What's the single most important thing I can do to survive with my Restless Legs Syndrome (RLS)?

   Answer: Practice *zero tolerance*. This means you use a safe and reliable method to stop it as quickly as possible. If this means walking, then walk. Do not let the sensations build. You can expand your arsenal of safe and reliable responses later.

2. Is there a drug that works for RLS?

   Answer: Many prescription medications are prescribed to help with RLS. Some medicines target chemical imbalances, while others help induce sleep or calm the mind or body. While this book was being written, the FDA approved a drug, Requip, to be used for RLS. The drug was already being used for Parkinson's patients, but new trials showed it could be useful with RLS cases. Of course, this does not mean it works for all RLSers, or that it is without undesirable side effects. For more information, see the chapter "Prop Tricks: Prescription."

3. Why should I use a Bag of Tricks when I can just take a pill and get relief?

   Answer: The use of prescription medications for RLS relief can be extremely complicated. It is seldom a matter of finding one pill and getting all the relief you expect. In many cases, people end up dealing with "drug cocktails" (multiple drugs), and "drug holidays" (breaks from drugs which become ineffective or create side effects after long-term use). There are many other problems with relying on one medication as your only therapy for RLS. These problems are covered in later chapters of the book.

4. Will my RLS get worse with age?

Answer: Though people tend to complain more about their RLS symptoms as they get older and the symptoms seem to increase in severity and frequency, there's no proof of anything that has degenerated or progressed, physically, to cause more RLS as we age. This question is addressed in the previous chapter "RLS Basics."

5. Should I find an RLS specialist to treat me?

Answer: If there is an RLS specialist in your area, you can try that route. However, it's possible you will be just as well off with any doctor you think is open-minded, ready to learn, and willing to share information with you. Just as there isn't one treatment that works for everyone, there isn't one type of doctor that is best. Rather than looking for a specialist, search for a special doctor who is willing to be an active member of your RLS survival program.

RLS and Periodic Limb Movement Disorder (PLMD)

PERIODIC LIMB MOVEMENT Disorder (PLMD) is closely related to RLS. PLMD causes multiple involuntary jerking movements while a person sleeps. This book focuses on prevention and relief of RLS symptoms. If it brings corresponding positive results to PLMD symptoms, that is a bonus. The following is a list of important differences between RLS and PLMD:

1. **Diagnosis:** There is no clinical test for RLS. It is diagnosed by asking certain questions about a person's symptoms. PLMD can be accurately diagnosed through a sleep study or unofficially identified by having your sleep partner observe what happens when you are asleep.

2. **Sleep vs. awake:** RLS symptoms occur while you are awake and aware of feeling irresistible urges to move. PLMD movements happen while you are sleeping and usually unaware of your movements. The involuntary jerking movements can occur several times in a minute. Sleeping partners of people with PLMD are the ones who are aware of the movements and complain the most about their sleep being interrupted. There are cases of "daytime PLMD," but I will not complicate the issue by going into that now.

3. **Voluntary vs. Involuntary movements:** Irresistible urges lead RLSers to make voluntary movements. There are some cases of involuntary jerking attributed to RLS, but they are not typically characteristic of the syndrome. If you insist your movements are involuntary (because you have to move to avoid going crazy), consider the following analogy. If someone put a gun to your head and said, "Move, or I'll shoot!" you would have to move in order to avoid being shot. Though it wouldn't seem like you had much choice, you would be moving voluntarily. By contrast, if the sudden shock and the presence of the gun made you jump before you had time to think or take deliberate action, your movement would be involuntary.

4. **Preventing sleep vs. Disturbing sleep:** RLS symptoms can prevent you from getting to sleep. After a night of RLS symptoms, you will know you did not get enough sleep. With PLMD, people think they get a good night's sleep, but their jerking prevents them from ever reaching a restorative stage of sleep. They probably wonder why they feel so exhausted, even though they slept for so long.

5. **Variables affecting RLS and PLMD:** RLS symptoms can be triggered by many variables, including coexisting ailments, foods, deficiencies, and physical surroundings. We can change these variables and notice differences in our RLS symptoms. Since PLMD occurs during sleep, it is hard to make similar correlations between adjustments of aggravating variables and changes in periodic limb movements. We could add vitamins or eliminate aggravating foods, but without repeating a sleep study, it would be hard to show a decrease in PLMD symptoms. Though it is believed that approximately 80 percent of RLSers also have PLMD, we are not sure how the two conditions are connected. Since so many who have one

tend to have the other, there is a good chance the variables affecting the two are similar.

6. **Relief obtained in RLS and PLMD:** If the same variables affect RLS and PLMD, it makes sense to expect some of the treatments for RLS to relieve PLMD symptoms. If an RLS treatment helps a person get to sleep without urges to squirm, we can hope the same treatment would help that person stay still while sleeping. Many RLSers have used the RLS Rebel Program and reported improvements in their PLMD. Their reports were based on feelings of being more rested during the day, even though they did not have clinical proof of decreased periodic limb movements during sleep.

Quick Start Tips

'M OFTEN ASKED, "If there were only one thing you could recommend for dealing with Restless Legs Syndrome (RLS), what would it be?"

My answer is always, "If you do nothing else, use *zero tolerance*. Do not tolerate it. Stop it the minute it starts."

If you are experiencing an RLS attack right now or have an understandable impatience and need some fast answers before you will be able to read this book in detail, consider the following Quick Start Tips. Most importantly, apply the first tip—*zero tolerance*. Whether you have to walk, use a prescription medication, or totally avoid an RLS-provoking activity, do your best to avoid or stop any RLS attacks immediately. You can perfect your methods and bolster your stores of ammunition later. Right now, you need to "get a grip." I hope the following tips will tide you over and give you that grip until you can sit still and read the rest of this book.

1. **Practice *zero tolerance*.** Stop an RLS attack as soon as it starts. Kick the mattress, stretch, or get up and walk. Do whatever it takes to stop it, at least temporarily. Do not let RLS symptoms escalate. The faster you stop them, the easier it will be to apply your planned tricks. If you let it build up for a while, it only gets harder to control.

2. **Become an RLS rebel.** Refuse to be a helpless victim. Decide to fight back.

3. **Decide to work hard at surviving with RLS.** Accept the fact there is currently no cure for RLS. Realize there are no easy answers. Whether you use prescription medications or alternative methods, you will continually be adjusting dosages, rotating treatments, and dealing with changes in your RLS symptoms. It is definitely possible to reduce the severity and frequency of RLS, but it won't be an easy task. Become educated about RLS and work as a team with your doctor to improve your survival skills.

4. **Count on it.** Plan on the *RLS bully* always being there when you try to be still. It makes more sense to expect it to show up and to be prepared with positive ways to respond (tricks) than to wish it would not show up and then be shocked, unprepared, and victimized. Why not be prepared and just count on it showing up when you hop into bed tonight?

5. **Call it a bully, not a beast.** Resist a victimized attitude and adopt an attitude of empowerment. Learn to reduce the *beast of RLS* to bully size, where you can manage it more successfully. The Reduction Plan will guide you in ways to reduce the *beast of RLS*. Develop confidence in your responses to RLS attacks. Feeling victimized only leads to panic, which leads to fear, which leads to anxiety, which makes your RLS worse. If you are unsuccessful with your treatments one night, make adjustments in the morning and try again the next night. You will soon become a confident and skilled RLS rebel. Before long, you will realize you are much tougher than the *RLS bully*.

6. **Eliminate the aggravators.** Analyze anything that might aggravate your RLS attacks. Consider the effects of caffeine products, antihistamines, and medications. Medicines that are initially used to control RLS can also start aggravating it. There are reports that some anti-nausea, anti-psychotic, and anti-depressant drugs will aggravate RLS. Lack

of sleep is an aggravator, too. RLS symptoms may worsen when you need to get going on projects (e.g., paying bills, planning events). For some folks, overeating will trigger RLS symptoms.

7. **Plan your responses.** Don't wait for an RLS attack to start before you begin wondering how to respond. You need to have a plan. This is where the Bag of Tricks Approach (BOTA) comes in. You may need a choice of plans, depending on the type of RLS attack and the situation you are trying to endure. For instance, if the RLS feelings have caused knotted muscles, you might need walking, stretching, or deep massage. If you have squirmy feelings in your legs or arms, you might need a quick walk or a little exercise. If you are experiencing an overall body attack and are filled with panic and a desire to escape, you might need a hot bath or brisk walk, followed by a special herbal tea and a good mind-consuming computer game. Learn to react to symptoms quickly and aggressively, with planned and appropriate responses.

8. **Minimize the panic.** Though RLS attacks may return over and over again, it is important to remember they will eventually stop. RLS is not fatal. The goal is to stop it immediately. Replace panic and ignorance with knowledge, self-analysis, and a Plan of Attack.

Don't waste energy worrying about whether your RLS will get worse. Spend your time and energy learning effective ways to prevent the majority of symptoms. For symptoms that insist on occurring, be ready with fast and reliable tricks. It takes time to perfect skills that will help you become a confident RLS rebel.

It's time to
GET EDUCATED,
FIGHT BACK, *and*
TAKE CONTROL!

The RLS Rebel Program

Restless Legs Syndrome (RLS) is an elusive syndrome. Treatments may work for one person, but not for the next. They may work this time, but not next time. We may be able to sit through a movie tonight, but not tomorrow. When dealing with RLS, we can easily become confused and frustrated, not knowing where to begin or how to proceed. Many RLSers run out of ideas to try and do not know where to turn. We need something to help us get the most out of our treatments and keep our strategies organized, reliable, and effective.

The solution to our need for organization and direction is the RLS Rebel Program. It is a comprehensive organizational program, designed to help RLSers manage their RLS survival. It is also the simplest answer to the question: How do you survive with RLS? It is a *one-size-fits-all*, personalized, organizational approach, allowing the RLSer to remain empowered.

An organizational approach

The RLS Rebel Program was developed in 2001 as a way to help RLSers and their supporters recognize all the areas that must be considered when dealing with RLS. The program encourages RLSers to address two main areas. First, we must reduce the *beast of RLS*, turning it into a mere *RLS bully*. This is accomplished by using the six steps of the Reduction Plan. Next, we must apply a combination of tricks in a systematic approach. This is achieved by skillful application of the four steps of the Bag of Tricks Approach (BOTA).

The core of the RLS Rebel Program is its two-part outline, listing the steps of the Reduction Plan and the BOTA. In the following chapter, I will explain how the outline can be used to develop a file system that will organize all the parts of your RLS Rebel Program. Your file system will allow you to relax, knowing you have everything you need, right at your fingertips.

One size fits all, but still personalized

How can a one-size-fits-all program work for a syndrome that is so varied, and how can a generic program be personalized? The RLS Rebel Program is merely a guideline, pointing out areas each RLSer needs to address. It becomes personalized as you fill in those areas with your unique information.

This book provides information and ideas to get you started on the RLS Rebel Program. It is up to each person to log results of treatments, add new treatment ideas, list questions to research, or decide what parts of the program to apply. Each person's RLS rebel program will follow the same outline, but will contain totally different information from anyone else's program.

The only exception

Though the RLS Rebel Program can be used by all RLSers, not all RLSers will embrace the program. It is for people who are determined to fight back and to stay in charge of their RLS survival methods. The program requires RLSers to stay actively involved by continuously addressing the various parts of the program. The RLSer makes the decisions, analyzes the results, and develops the changes that will bring about improved results.

An example of an RLSer who might not embrace the RLS Rebel Program is a lady who said to me, "Your program is just fine, Jill, but at my age, as severe as my RLS is, and after all the years I have struggled with it, I deserve an easier solution."

After asking a few questions, I found out she was five years younger than me, she had RLS only in her legs, and she experienced it only when she tried going to sleep. I was having it any time of day, every day, and in arms and legs. She had been dealing with RLS symptoms for only four years, whereas I had dealt with it for more than forty.

The RLS Rebel Program might have fit this lady, but I don't think the lady fit the RLS Rebel Program. A victimized, helpless attitude will not work with the RLS Rebel Program. You must have rebellious attitudes, determination, and perseverance. You must believe you can take charge of your life, despite the obnoxious *RLS bully*.

Understand the program's benefits

The RLS Rebel Program's advantages make it useful to all RLSers, regardless of their choice of treatments, the variables influencing their RLS, or the severity of their symptoms.

1. **All treatments are possible.** The program eliminates the *drugs versus alternatives* debate, because all treatments can be considered and used. At any point in the survival program, an RLSer may decide to use prescription medications, alternative methods, self-help methods, or a combination of several methods.

2. **The combination approach insures success.** The BOTA avoids the futility of trying to rely on one pill or therapy to handle everything. When a person has the flexibility to choose the best tricks for the current situation, success becomes a reasonable expectation.

3. **Flexibility insures longevity.** Adjustments are continually needed due to changes in an RLSer's age, improvement in survival skills, occurrence of apparent remissions, or the onset of new aggravators (e.g., an injury, surgery, coexisting ailment). The program encourages flexibility and change, making it a program that can be useful throughout an RLSer's life.

4. **Treatment priorities are addressed easily.** The RLS Rebel program adapts to all priorities and allows flexibility when those priorities change. Today, the priority might be to catch up on sleep. Later, the priority could change to a need to sit still through a meeting, lecture, or long airplane trip.

Let's get started

By reading this survival guide, you have already started the RLS Rebel Program. How you proceed with it is totally up to you. Remember, it is your program, guided by you and designed to fit your needs. The following are suggestions for how to continue developing your own program:

1. **Take notes and make highlights.** Unless a cure is found, you will use the information in this survival guide for many years. I suggest you make notes in the margins, highlight important parts, and make separate notes in your file system. Make this your personal training guide, adding comments that pertain to you and your RLS survival.

2. **Survey the layout.** It is always a good idea to familiarize yourself with the layout or organization of a book. This is especially important if you plan to use the book as a quick reference. By studying the Table of Contents, you will notice that details of the RLS Rebel Program Outline are described in Part I: The Reduction Plan and Part II:

The BOTA. The chapters in these two sections will be the foundation for developing your RLS Rebel Program.

3. **You can start filing now.** If you are in a hurry to develop your RLS program, you can start your file system before reading the rest of this survival guide. Begin by reading the next chapter and following its suggestions. As you read the subsequent chapters, you can begin filing your notes and writing your personal plan of action for each section of the RLS Rebel Program.

4. **Share the program.** I suggest you share this survival guide, using the format and terminology as a basis for communicating with your supporters. Whether your supporters are family, friends, healthcare providers, or support group leaders, it will help if they understand your approach to RLS. Show your supporters the two chapters in the last section of this book that were written specifically for those who support RLSers ("To Our RLS Healthcare Providers" and "To Those Who Support Us").

The RLS Rebel Program Outline

THE RLS REBEL Program Outline is the core of the RLS Rebel Program. The program was developed to deal with every possible aspect of surviving with Restless Legs Syndrome (RLS). The outline was developed to organize all those aspects. Everything you need to remember, consider, or include in your RLS program can be filed into one of the sections of the outline.

When I first presented the RLS Rebel Program, the outline was merely a public speaking tool for organizing my lecture. The catchy titles, such as Reduce Panic, Reduce Chaos, and Pack Your Bags, were put on poster boards and used as attention-getting props. Later, I realized the outline could be a valuable tool for RLSers. It makes perfect delineations for a file system that organizes our RLS information, our logs of what we have done, and our plans for the future.

The section titles have the added benefit of being easy to memorize. After routine use of the RLS Rebel Program Outline, RLSers can easily recall the outline's catchy titles. As each section is reviewed, the outline becomes a useful checklist for monitoring RLS survival programs.

The RLS Rebel Program Outline has two parts. In Part I: The Reduction Plan, there are six steps that help reduce the *beast of RLS*, turning it into a mere *RLS bully*. In Part II: The Bag of Tricks Approach (BOTA), we gather and apply a combination of tricks in a systematic approach.

PART I: The REDUCTION PLAN
    Step 1: Reduce PANIC
    (Get educated)
    Step 2: Reduce CHAOS
    (Analyze symptoms)
    Step 3: Reduce SYMPTOMS
    (Identify coexisting ailments)
    Step 4: Reduce DEFICIENCIES
    (Adjust supplements)
    Step 5: Reduce AGGRAVATORS
    (Identify triggers)
    Step 6: Reduce SITUATIONS
    (Prioritize needs)

PART II: The BAG OF TRICKS APPROACH (BOTA)
    Step 1: GATHER YOUR TRICKS
    (List all treatment options)
    Step 2: PACK YOUR BAGS
    (Match treatments with activities)
    Step 3: PLAN OF ATTACK
    (Your plan for getting through an activity)
    Step 4: RELIEF PLANS
    (Your plan to stop symptoms, immediately)

Develop a file system

The best way to use the RLS Rebel Program is to set up a file system in which you keep all your RLS survival information. It can be a file folder system, a divided three-ring notebook, or a computer directory with multiple folders. Personally, I like the portability and flexibility of a hard copy system like a three-ring notebook. Here are some tips for developing and using your file system:

1. **Use the RLS Rebel Program Outline's catchy titles to label sections of your file system.** You can use the titles from each section of the RLS Rebel Program Outline to

label your folders or the various sections of your note-book. You should have six sections for the Reduction Plan and four sections for the BOTA.

2. **Make it a habit to file new information.** Keep all your RLS information in this file system. As you come across new information, articles, or newsletters you want to save, train yourself to add them to the appropriate sections of your file system. If you change your medications, record the changes in your file system. If you keep blank paper in each section, you can easily record your notes. For already-printed information, there are several options for filing. If you use a notebook system, you can get pocketed dividers or clear plastic sleeves to hold extra material or you can punch holes in the printed material and add it directly to the notebook. If you use a file folder system, just drop the information in the correct folder. If you use a computer file system, you may have to scan the information before adding it to your computer files. You might also be able to find a copy of the article online and just transfer that information to your files.

3. **Identify new material.** As you add articles or new information to your files, be sure to record the source of the information. It takes only a minute to write a date and the name of the magazine or website URL before storing the information in your file system.

4. **Keep a contents cover sheet at the start of each section.** At the front of each section, keep a list or log of what you add to that section. If you number each entry of the log, you can put a corresponding number on the top right corner of the information pertaining to that entry and then place that information in chronological order with what is already in the file. Later, if you are looking for information about an RLS study or a certain drug or

therapy you tried, you can scan the cover list, find the number of the article or page you need, and flip straight to the right spot.

5. **Keep a history and a "Things to Try" list.** Record as much as you can about everything you try. You can keep information about your doctors, drugs, supplements, and aggravators. You can comment on what worked, what didn't work, and what adjustments you made. If you come across ideas you can't try immediately, store those ideas in the appropriate section and title them, "Things to Try." If someone gives you a new therapy idea or mentions an article you should read, make a note of it in the appropriate section and the idea will be saved until you are ready to pursue it. If you suddenly feel as if you are out of ideas, you can check your "Things to Try" list. You can also review your histories, and see if there is something that did not work the first time but might work now.

Why wait?

You may find it useful to set up your file system before progressing further in this survival guide. As you read the following chapters, you can start adding information and making notes to yourself about things to try. These notes can immediately go into their appropriate sections and be easy to locate when needed.

RLS REBEL PROGRAM

Part I: The Reduction Plan

Understanding
the Reduction Plan

What are we reducing?

FOR MANY RLSERS, symptoms begin in childhood, when we have difficulty being still during long car trips or when watching television, sitting in school, or getting to sleep. When we complain or seek professional help, we are told, "It's just growing pains." As we get older, our symptoms become more irritating and more disruptive during our at-rest activities. Without even realizing it, we begin avoiding certain situations where Restless Legs Syndrome (RLS) is likely to occur. Before we know it, the *beast of RLS* is out of control and has totally disturbed our lives. At this point, even strong medications may not help, because the *beast of RLS* is fueled by too many variables and has become entirely out of control. The six steps of the Reduction Plan address the six main variables whose constant management will result in reducing the out-of-control *beast of RLS* and maintaining him as a mere *RLS bully*.

Why do we reduce before we treat?

If we knew the cause of RLS, we could probably just treat for it and be done. As it is, we must look at the variables we have identified as making RLS symptoms worse. If we can adjust those variables and reduce the size and impact of the *beast of RLS*, it will be easier to treat the remaining symptoms. If you had an infected sore, you would clean it out and minimize the area you needed to treat with antibiotics and ointments. By reducing the *beast of RLS* to a manageable size, it is as though we are cleaning up the sore. Once we are dealing with a reduced beast (a mere *RLS bully*), we will be able to achieve better results from whatever combination of treatments we use.

Why do we repeat the Reduction Plan?

The variables affecting our RLS and the treatments we choose seldom stay the same. We must constantly review the various sections of the RLS Rebel Program Outline and note changes in our lives that might affect our RLS experience. If the RLSer is maintaining a file system, with a section for each of the steps of the Reduction Plan, it will become a simple task to keep track of new information, review old information, and record new strategies, questions, or theories. There are several reasons to constantly repeat and review the Reduction Plan.

1. **New information.** Information about RLS changes quickly. My initial notes on RLS said it did not occur in children. Later that year, RLS literature began citing many cases of childhood RLS. In my original manuscript for this book, I stated there were no FDA approved medicines for RLS. Before I finished editing the manuscript, the FDA approved the first drug for RLS. Never assume you have completed your RLS education. By staying abreast of current RLS information, you can continue to reduce your *RLS bully*.

2. **New ailments.** Occasionally question whether the nature or severity of your RLS symptoms has changed. New, coexisting ailments could be complicating your RLS. If so, it would make sense to treat those ailments before treating the aggravated RLS symptoms. Always

expect your physical health to change and create new reasons to review steps of the Reduction Plan.

3. **New aggravators.** New medications, changes in your lifestyle, or changes in your diet, can create new variables to reduce. Something may not have bothered you last week, but might become an aggravator of your RLS, this week.

4. **Better results this time.** Some adjustments do not appear to make a difference when they are first tried. A person with out-of-control RLS might find the elimination of caffeine makes no apparent difference in RLS symptoms. Later, after that same person removes other aggravating variables, the elimination of caffeine might produce noticeably positive results.

When bullies become beasts

When an *RLS bully* suddenly reverts to being the *beast of RLS*, there is often an obvious reason for the change. I have known people to review sections of their Reduction Plan and realize they started using a product which they had previously listed as an aggravator, but had forgotten to avoid. Others have discovered their RLS was being aggravated by another ailment, which the doctor quickly diagnosed and treated. Once that ailment was treated, the *beast of RLS* was once again reduced to an *RLS bully*. The *beast of RLS* will always try to take over. When he does, review the Reduction Plan, and turn him right back into the bully he really is.

Step 1: Reduce Panic

(Get educated)

PANIC CAN EASILY aggravate your RLS. Panic is generated by fear, and fear is generated by the unknown. Therefore, the best way to reduce panic is to get educated.

Gather as much information as possible about RLS, RLS treatments, and your healthcare options. In this section of your file system, you might keep contact information about your doctor, support groups, or pharmacy. You might keep lists of favorite websites and books on RLS. This section can be the perfect spot to hold articles, newsletters, or even videos and other recordings from conferences on RLS. Never stop gathering RLS information.

Directories and referrals

Use this section to record healthcare providers' phone numbers, addresses, fax numbers, office hours, names of office personnel, and any other pertinent contact information.

If you hear of a new doctor you might want to visit in the future, write down the contact information in this section. You can staple or tape business cards to the pages if you are keeping a notebook or file folder system, or you can include links to a doctor's website if you are keeping your file system on the computer.

You may want to collect lists of recommended RLS doctors and note which ones are preferred by your insurance plan. You can use this section to list health insurance information that could affect the coverage of your RLS treatments.

The Internet

It is risky to list Internet sites in a book, because they are constantly changing. I have listed some useful sites that have been in existence and actively maintained for several years. Use them to expand your growing knowledge of RLS.

The RLS Rebel Program:
http://rlsrebel.com

> This is the official website of the RLS Rebel. The site is similar to, but less extensive than, this book. The website has fun pictures, more humor, and some of my first thoughts and articles on dealing with RLS.

The Restless Legs Syndrome Foundation:
http://www.rls.org

> This website is an absolute must for anyone researching RLS. See the comments below about membership in the RLS Foundation and how to receive their quarterly newsletter, *Nightwalkers*. Along with information about RLS, the website has access to an RLS chat group and discussion board, RLS publications, and links to important RLS websites.

Southern California RLS Support Group Website:
http://www.rlshelp.org

> This extensive website includes an archive of letters and experiences shared by members of a real-time support group that meets in the Los Angeles/Orange County area. The site is maintained by their advisor, Dr. Mark J. Buchfuhrer, and has one of the largest lists

of alternative treatment ideas, including medical com-mentary on many.

Cyberspace Email Support Group: http://groups.yahoo.com

If you are not already a member of yahoo.com, you will have to do the free sign up. Once you are into the "groups" section, do a search for "rlssupport." This will take you to a group with more than 1,000 members who have a collective wealth of knowledge and experience. Sign up for the digest version and you will receive only one daily email of all the newest letters.

RLS books

Until 2005, I recommended that every RLSer and medical professional treating RLS get their hands on a copy of *Sleep Thief*, by Virginia Wilson. This book documented research, medical opinions, and reports from RLSers prior to 1996. It is still one of the best compilations of medical and lay information on RLS. It also provides an excellent history of various RLS events, including the formation of the RLS Foundation.

In 2005, coinciding with the first FDA approval of an RLS medicine, several books were authored by well-respected doctors and authorities in the RLS field. The books (including this one) were due for publication in 2006. Some were directed to medical professionals, while others were directed to RLSers. By checking publication dates, you should be able to identify the newest books.

Be aware, there are several publications with catchy titles that lead you to believe their pages hold the answer to a cure—but remember, if a cure is found, you will probably hear about it on the news or from the RLS Foundation. I'm sure you will hear about it faster than someone could write a book and get it published. Be leery of titles that promise too much.

Organizations

Each year, more and more organizations and groups become interested in Restless Legs Syndrome. There are many groups doing research, conducting studies, and putting out valuable educational material about RLS. These groups include the National Institute of Health (NIH), the Restless Legs Syndrome Foundation, and various sleep organizations and drug companies. Check their websites, and keep yourself informed.

The RLS Foundation is probably the most important organization for RLSers to monitor. I highly recommend every RLSer become a member of the RLS Foundation. As a member, you will receive the latest RLS information in their quarterly newsletter, "Nightwalkers." You can keep your newsletters filed in this section (Reduce Panic) of your file system. The RLS Foundation will also be happy to send RLS information to your doctors and to support you in starting an RLS support group.

If you do not have computer access to the link, above, you can contact the RLS Foundation at:

Restless Legs Syndrome Foundation, Inc.
819 Second Street SW
Rochester MN 55902-2985
email: rlsfoundation@rls.org
Phone: (507) 287-6465
FAX: (507) 287-6312

Support groups and other gatherings

RLS support groups are in nearly every state of the United States. They also exist in several other countries. They are usually organized by volunteer leaders who have RLS and have received information and support from the RLS Foundation. Some groups have medical advisors. Guest speakers often provide information at meetings. One of the great benefits of any support group comes from being able to share experiences and learn from others who understand. The RLS Foundation's newsletter lists websites and contact information for many support groups. You can also find that information at the RLS Foundation website: http://www.rls.org.

The RLS Foundation conducts yearly meetings and conferences around the country. Other organizations have similar workshops, seminars, or conferences, geared to their own focus, but including RLS in their material and presentations. Be on the lookout for and consider attending sessions about sleep disorders, movement disorders, or other ailments and conditions known to aggravate RLS symptoms. It can be very helpful to attend events that focus on nutrition, stress, exercise, emotional health, or other issues that can affect RLS. By learning more about how to insure good sleep and how to control other aggravating conditions, you will indirectly be fighting your RLS.

Step 2: Reduce Chaos

(Analyze symptoms)

Our first experiences with Restless Legs Syndrome (RLS) may seem chaotic. Many RLSers do not know when their symptoms will appear, what makes them worse, or what treatments bring relief. It is not uncommon to hear people say, "I never know when it will hit" or "I have no way to stop it once it starts."

When we closely examine our RLS attacks, they become less chaotic and more predictable as we discover patterns, behaviors, and tendencies. We can begin analyzing our RLS by asking, "What works?" and "What does not work?"

What works?

Walking, mental distraction, and stretching are responses that will stop an RLS attack, at least temporarily. Though RLSers often complain about having to walk, walking is really a blessing. It is our handiest and most effective response to RLS. Granted, we would be happier if we didn't have to walk, but if you consider the situations where RLSers do not have the option to walk (e.g., in cases of paralysis, recovering from surgery, being in an airplane with the seat belt sign on), you will quickly realize what a blessing it is to be able to walk and relieve RLS symptoms.

We also know that mental distraction can be a very effective response. By getting into a heated discussion or focusing on something in a movie (e.g., counting how many times a person says a certain word or how many times they blink), we can sometimes create enough mental distraction to overpower the urges to move.

Stretching is especially important when the irresistible urges progress to knotted muscles. Excessive physical movements (e.g., 100 heel lifts) can also tire the limbs and make them want to be still. However, too much physical exercise right before an at-rest activity will worsen some people's RLS symptoms.

Many RLSers actually find their best response to RLS symptoms is to go to sleep quickly. For most of my life, RLS tended to hit when I was very tired. If I could just fall asleep, even for ten minutes, I would wake up without symptoms and be able to sit still. It was later in life, in my forties, when RLS symptoms started interfering with my ability to fall asleep.

What does not work?

Trying to ignore your RLS symptoms or telling yourself to just sit still, usually will not work. Although, I have been known to tell myself, "Everything is fine. You are not going anywhere and there is no danger, so just relax and focus on something." Sometimes it works, but it is never a reliable response. Slowly relaxing from toe to head usually makes RLS symptoms worse. Trying to be still so as to not disturb your sleep partner or the person next to you at the movies only makes things worse. Ironically, these responses constitute the strategy most RLSers use before they finally learn about RLS and develop a useful response plan. It is no wonder they think of their symptoms as chaotic and panic when the symptoms suddenly appear.

Describe it, predict it, and treat it

As you observe and analyze your RLS symptoms, make notes in this section of your filing system. Describe what works, what does not work, when the symptoms are likely to appear, and what types of symptoms appear in each situation. You may find you get the crawly feelings in your arms when you are reading, but when you are watching TV the feelings are followed by knotted thigh muscles.

Once you have described your RLS symptoms, you will be able to predict when and how they will appear. You will also be able to prepare the best responses or prevention methods for each situation. When I began recording my observations and making predictions about my own RLS, I recorded some of the following comments:

> "It tends to be worse in the evenings, when watching TV, at movie theaters, when I am a passenger in a car, and when I am wearing confining clothing."

> "I tend to have two or three very bad RLS nights each month, exactly ten days after the start of my menstrual cycle."

> "My RLS attacks are worse when I am about to start a new project or need to get going on something, like paying my bills. My symptoms are less bothersome once I am involved in the project."

> "My RLS tends to show up in four different forms:
>
> 1. Crawly, irresistible urges to move my legs.
> 2. Irresistible urges to move my arms.
> 3. Leg urges, followed by a hardening or knotting of thigh muscles.
> 4. Overall body panic; wanting to shake my whole body and flee from weird web-like feelings."

Once you realize your RLS symptoms vary, you can adjust the treatments according to the type of RLS you are facing. When you realize there is a pattern or a certain amount of predictability, you can plan your responses in advance or avoid situations where the RLS would normally show up.

**If you can describe it, you can predict it.
If you can predict it, you can treat it.**

Step 3: Reduce Symptoms

(Identify coexisting ailments)

IN STEP 2 of the Reduction Plan (Reduce Chaos), you learned to identify and predict the main symptom of Restless Legs Syndrome (RLS), irresistible urges to move. RLSers may complain of other problems, including pain, exhaustion, insomnia, burning sensations, or tingling. Though some of these additional symptoms can be a direct result of RLS, there is also a chance they are being caused by coexisting ailments. When two or more ailments produce similar symptoms, treatment strategies may become complicated and progress might be hard to detect. In Step 3: Reduce Symptoms, you will identify coexisting ailments that may be responsible for aggravating or causing some of the symptoms previously associated only with RLS.

The complications of dealing with coexisting ailments can be visualized if you make an imaginary pile of all symptoms and complaints associated with your RLS (e.g., irresistible urges to move, exhaustion, pain, depression, tingling sensations, insomnia, anxiety, restlessness). Add to the imaginary pile all the symptoms you experience from other ailments (e.g., arthritis, fibromyalgia, stress, mental disorders, diabetes, back injuries). You may find yourself adding a symptom to the pile more than once if that symptom is shared by more than one ailment. For example, if you have arthritis, fibromyalgia, and RLS, you might add *exhaustion* and *pain* several times.

Once you have loaded the pile with all the symptoms from your RLS and your co-existing ailments, add all the treatments you use for each ailment and symptom. Include pain medications, sleeping aids, exercise, diet, herbal teas, or whatever else you do to address various complaints. Finally, top off the pile with all the results you would expect from your treatments (e.g., no urges to move, less pain, relief of tingling, more energy, a feeling of being rested). Looking at your pile, can you make sense of your situation? Can you tell which symptoms belong with which ailments and which treatments relieve which symptoms?

By now, your imaginary pile should look like a management nightmare and a perfect breeding ground for the *beast of RLS*. By reducing the huge messy pile of symptoms, ailments and treatments to an organized record of symptoms and their appropriate treatments, you will keep the *beast of RLS* reduced to bully size.

Identify coexisting ailments

In this section of your notebook, list all the symptoms associated with your RLS (e.g., exhaustion, pain, depression, an inability to sit still). Next, work with your doctor to identify other ailments that might trigger the same symptoms. The exhaustion, pain, or tingling you thought were RLS symptoms might actually be caused by lower back problems, peripheral neuropathy, diabetes, sleep apnea, or Periodic Limb Movement Disorder (PLMD).

With your doctor, decide what ailments and symptoms should be treated first. For instance, if you suffer from exhaustion, it might make sense to treat a coexisting case of sleep apnea or PLMD, rather than treating RLS. If you treat only for RLS, you might still be exhausted from the sleep apnea and PLMD.

If your RLS tricks have been reliable for a long time but suddenly stop working effectively, do not assume your RLS is getting worse. You might be experiencing the worsening of another ailment and its symptoms, which also happen to be symptoms shared by RLS. If so, you will want to treat that ailment, rather than assuming your RLS is worse or thinking you need to increase the dosage of an RLS treatment.

As you are considering coexisting ailments, keep an eye out for other triggers that can aggravate RLS symptoms. Medications are especially prone to produce side effects that mimic symptoms. You might find a way to calm your urges to move and even sleep through the night, but a medication may leave you exhausted, despite your extra sleep.

Target symptoms with specific treatments

By carefully isolating symptoms, you can begin targeting treatments to specific symptoms. As you list your treatments, make a note about the results and side effects you can expect from each treatment. One treatment may relieve multiple symptoms. A pain medication may relieve pain and have an extra benefit of inducing sleep.

One of my favorite RLS distraction tricks is to suck on my favorite brand of sucker. This trick is effective against the symptom of irresistible urges to squirm (caused by RLS), but it will not help with exhaustion (caused by sleep deprivation), tingling feet (caused by peripheral neuropathy), or sore joints (caused by arthritis). Those symptoms need to be addressed with other treatments.

Create a visual representation

The notes you make in this section of your notebook will help you manage and visually represent your symptoms, ailments, and treatments. Be as creative as you want, making lists, charts, or other visuals that will help you represent your situation. For instance, you can make a simple chart with four columns: the first column listing symptoms, the second column listing the ailments you think are responsible for those symptoms, the third column listing the treatments being used to alleviate the symptoms, and the fourth column listing the results or side effects of the treatments.

You could also develop a rating system, giving each symptom a number that represents how important it is to treat it. Insomnia might rate a 10, meaning it's a high priority for treatment. Pain that is mild and intermittent might rate a 2, meaning it's not a treatment issue.

Consider using your lists and charts to facilitate discussions with your doctor. Imagine showing your doctor a chart where the problem of sitting still at work was highlighted in red (high priority), but the symptom of getting to sleep was in pale yellow (low priority). There would be no question about your treatment priorities and the need for a treatment to help you sit still.

Communicate concisely and accurately

Dealing with more than one ailment, syndrome, or treatment, creates a real challenge to doctor-patient communication. If you walk into your doctor's office and complain of a long list of confusing symptoms, the doctor will have to sort through what you say and then determine which symptoms need to be treated first. The lists and notes you make while completing Step 3 of the Reduction Plan will facilitate concise and accurate communication between you and your doctor.

There's a riddle that asks, "How do you eat an elephant?" The answer is, "One bite at a time." If we were to apply that to RLS, we might ask, "How to you reduce the *beast of RLS*?" And we might answer, "One symptom at a time."

By reducing the huge messy pile of symptoms and ailments to a manageable record of your situation and by clearly communicating your priorities and treatments preferences, you and your doctor can keep the *beast of RLS* reduced to bully size. For more tips on developing efficient and productive communications with your doctor, see the chapter "Do's and Don'ts for Dealing with Your Doctor."

Step 4: Reduce Deficiencies

(Adjust supplements)

MANY SUPPLEMENTS HAVE been reported as being helpful in reducing Restless Legs Syndrome to a manageable state. It is usually easier for people to use supplements than to assure they are receiving enough vitamins or minerals from their diet. Dietary changes for RLSers tend to be more successful for eliminating aggravators (Step 5 of the Reduction Plan) than for compensating for deficiencies.

There are two ways to approach possible deficiencies. One option is to work with your doctor and test for deficiencies. The other option is to carefully try various supplements, one at a time, and see if they reduce the frequency or severity of your RLS attacks. Even if your medical tests do not show a deficiency, you may still benefit from certain vitamin and mineral supplements. To be safe, I suggest you discuss the use of supplements with your doctor.

Test for ferritin and other deficiencies

Regular blood tests can check many things, including the free-flowing iron in your system. Special blood tests are needed to check two other iron related items, ferritin and transferrin. Without getting into detailed medical descriptions, I would describe ferritin as your storage of iron and transferrin has the mechanism for getting your iron from storage into the free-flowing, normally-tested iron. I am sure some doctors would cringe at that explanation, but it works for the purposes of this chapter. One of the best explanations I have heard is to think of the relationship between ferritin, transferrin, and iron, as a checking account system. Ferritin is the money you have stored in the checking account. The checks are the transferrin, which gets the money out and can change it into cash. Iron is the cash. You can have plenty of cash (iron), but not have enough savings (ferritin).

When you get the results of your ferritin level test, be sure you ask for the number of your ferritin level. Do not settle for hearing your ferritin is "in the normal range." Normal, depending on which lab you use, can range from 10-200ng/ml. Studies have shown a marked improvement in RLS symptoms when an RLSer's ferritin is raised to at least 50ng/ml. If someone tells me his ferritin level is 15ng/ml, I respond by saying, "Congratulations! At least you have something concrete to treat." Reduction in severity and frequency of RLS symptoms can be expected when iron supplements are used, raising low ferritin levels to at least 50ng/ml.

Ferritin levels are known to drop during pregnancy. RLS is also known to be bothersome during pregnancy. It makes sense that prenatal care often includes iron supplementation.

Before you try supplementing with iron, be sure to consult your doctor. Iron is one supplement which can cause severe problems if taken incorrectly or by people who have health issues that make iron supplementation inadvisable.

Another test that could be helpful is a B-12 blood test. Iron, B-12, and dopamine work together in our brains. An imbalance of any of these can trigger increased RLS symptoms. Some prescription medications can deplete a person's B-12. It is important to test for this whenever a deficiency is suspected. As with iron, however, a report of "normal" does not necessarily rule out the possibility of benefiting from B-

12 supplementation. Many RLSers have normal reports from their B-12 tests, but still report noticeable benefits from taking extra B vitamins.

Consider supplements

What helps one person does not necessarily help another, but when a group of people, sharing the same physical condition, tend to use many of the same supplements, it makes sense to consider what they are using. Many RLSers have sworn they experienced beneficial results from taking extra B vitamins, iron, folic acid, calcium, magnesium, or vitamin E. By researching and working with health and diet professionals, you will learn what supplements to try and how to take them carefully and efficiently.

Look for changes in deficiencies

Changes in age, health, diet, and lifestyle, can all change our deficiencies. For example, you may have had plenty of vitamin B five years ago, but due to long-term use of a prescription medicine, your vitamin B may have been depleted. If you are pregnant, you may experience pregnancy-related deficiencies or nutritional needs that require supplementation during pregnancy, but will return to normal after giving birth. Repeat this step of the Reduction Plan periodically to evaluate your current deficiencies and supplementation needs.

Be careful

When experimenting with supplements, whether they are vitamins, minerals, or herbs, do your homework. Look for information on the following:

1. What helps them absorb best?
2. What interferes with their absorption?

3. What interactions or contraindications might they have with other medications?

4. What would be considered harmful amounts?

5. What would be the symptoms of harmful amounts?

6. Is the cost within your means?

Be consistent

To be consistent, you have to keep your dosages, brand names, and time of supplementation constant. Brand X of a calcium supplement might work totally differently than Brand Z, even though the listed amounts of ingredients are identical. Changing the time of day you take a supplement can also affect its impact. If you always take a certain supplement in the morning before eating, keep to that plan. If you shift it to nighttime, consider that to be a change and do not make any other changes until you are sure the change in time of day made no difference.

Be slow to make changes

Make one change at a time. I set up my vitamins, minerals, and supplements for two weeks at a time. When I restock my supply, I allow one change. This can be a change in the brand or dosage, the elimination of something, or the addition of a new product. If the results seem good, I often keep the same setup for another two weeks, making sure I wasn't just having an easy two-week period.

Be careful of finances and miracle products

Do not associate cost with effectiveness. You do not have to spend a fortune on a specially prepared supplement just to find out if you need more of a certain vitamin or mineral. I find good results with brands I get at Wal-Mart and other discount stores, while other products are only available from health food stores. Stick to brand names you trust and try to spend as little as possible, unless you have reason to believe an expensive product is more effective.

Many people will claim their supplements or tonics will cure your RLS. Be very leery of these claims. I have been offered several "thirty-day, money-back" guarantees from salespeople who hoped I would try their miracle product and recommend it to other RLSers. I always explain that it is not unheard of to have a thirty-day period when RLS symptoms are relatively calm, so there would be no way to know if their product actually caused the improvement.

Once, when a salesperson relentlessly begged me to try what he was sure would cure my RLS, I said, "Give me the product at no charge for six months. If it works (i.e., if I have six months of no RLS symptoms), I'll pay for those six months, buy more, and recommend it to RLSers. If not, you'll pay the cost."

Interestingly enough, though he had assured me his product would work, he turned down my offer.

Remember what we know about RLS. It is different for everyone. In a later chapter, "Is It Worth a Try?" you will find a discussion on how to decide what ideas are worth the investment of your time, energy, emotions, and finances. The old adage applies: "If it sounds too good to be true, it probably is." If you follow the advice of this old saying, you may end up feeling a little skeptical or pessimistic, but you will not risk being gullible and having people take advantage of your sincere desire for relief.

Keep detailed records

Keep detailed records of dosages, brand names, and the forms of the supplements. It is not enough to write: "I tried calcium." Record the dosage, how often you took it, what brand it was, what else you were taking with it, and its form (e.g., calcium citrate, calcium carbonate, a blend with other supplements). You might also make a note of where you purchased the supplement and what you paid for it. That way, if you decide to continue using it, you will have shopping information at your fingertips.

Keep a "Things to Try" list

As you do your research, you will find many things you will want to try. If you follow the plan of trying only one thing at a time, you may not be able to try the new idea, right away. Go to this section of your file system and add the new ideas to your "Things to Try" list. I often receive suggestions from well meaning people who are sure they know what supplement will help me. My simple response is, "Thank you for that information. I will be sure to add that to my list of things to try."

While you are waiting for the results of your current trials, you can be researching the next choices from your list. Read up on the best ways to use the supplement, conflicts with prescription medicines, and any potentially negative side effects. If you are taking prescription medications, or if you have other ailments to consider, always check with your doctor. Remember, when your doctor asks what you are currently taking, be sure to share the list of your current supplements and discuss the next items on your "Things to Try" list.

Step 5: Reduce Aggravators

(Identify triggers)

WHEN I FIRST started researching Restless Legs Syndrome (RLS), there was little consensus among doctors and RLSers on what aggravated RLS symptoms. Through persistent searching and sharing, common aggravators have finally emerged. Some of the silliest suspicions have produced likely culprits.

I remember seeing a post in an RLS email support group, asking, "Can bucket seats aggravate RLS?" I thought it was the silliest idea I'd heard in a long time, until several others reported they had severe RLS attacks when in a car with bucket seats. Some of them also noticed they did not have RLS when they rode in a truck with a high bench seat. As you read this chapter, keep in mind the very thing that aggravates one person's RLS might be a useful treatment for another RLSer. Nothing seems to hold true for everyone, but everything is worth considering.

Antihistamines

Possibly the most agreed-upon aggravators of RLS symptoms are antihistamines. In RLS circles, products like Benadryl and Tylenol PM have bad reputations. If your RLS symptoms flare when your allergies are the worst, it could be you are using an antihistamine that is aggravating your RLS.

Prescription medications

Certain classes of medications have been known to aggravate RLS. Be suspicious of antidepressant, anti-seizure, antipsychotic, and anti-nausea medications. These are just some of the prescription medications which many RLSers have reported as aggravating their RLS. Not all medications in each category are a problem, and not all of these would be a problem for everyone with RLS. In fact, some of these are given as treatments for RLS. Do your research and consult with your doctor about the potential of your prescription medications aggravating your RLS.

RLS medications

Sadly, some medications which are initially effective in relieving RLS can suddenly start aggravating RLS symptoms. The aggravation of symptoms tends to start after long-term use of certain drugs or after a dosage is raised too high. Sinemet is a good example of a drug that can be used effectively for RLS, if kept at low dosages. When the dosage is raised too high, Sinemet can become an RLS aggravator. In many cases, when a drug appears to lose its effectiveness, dosages are raised, and then the RLSer experiences either rebound (a shorter time when each dose is effective) or augmentation (when the RLS symptoms begin attacking earlier in the day or in other parts of the body), making the RLS experience worse than it was before taking the medication. Once augmentation or rebound occurs, the patient must either take a drug holiday (temporarily avoiding that medication) or permanently stop using the medication.

Food and drink

Many RLSers report caffeine or chocolate aggravate their RLS. Some RLSers claim caffeine causes them to experience painful RLS symptoms. For some, it just keeps them awake too long, allowing RLS symptoms time to attack before they can doze off to sleep. Still others swear caffeine makes their RLS better.

Alcohol can be an aggravator. Though many people think it will help them sleep, it tends to cause a restlessness that invites RLS symptoms. Red wine, in particular, seems to aggravate symptoms in many RLSers.

Some RLSers have reported ice cream as an aggravator. Others claim it is not a matter of what they eat, but how much they eat. Overeating and feeling bloated will often trigger severe RLS symptoms.

Other aggravators

As you analyze your RLS behavior, look for anything that tends to trigger your attacks. There are obvious situations, like trying to sleep, sitting through a movie, or flying in an airplane. Also consider things like eating too much, eating foods that are too rich, wearing certain clothes (too restricting or not restricting enough), certain people and conversations, certain types of movies, reading magazines or television listings, having your bills and paperwork stack up, not accomplishing enough on a project with a deadline, exercise, and lack of exercise.

In this section of my file system, I have listed some specific observations of things that have been known to aggravate my RLS.

1. The tone of some people's voices and their slow manner of speaking.

2. Reading a television schedule, whether in a magazine or on the digital cable channel.

3. Silly movies where someone keeps getting deeper and deeper into trouble.

4. Any television show that keeps breaking for commercials and advertising what will happen when you return.

5. Reading magazines and catalogues.

6. Attending symphony concerts.

Knowing these are my RLS aggravators does not necessarily mean I avoid these activities. Instead, if I decide to do any of these, I take extra care to stop the RLS attacks as soon as they start and have my responses ready to use at a moment's notice.

Hospital warnings

If you are going to be a hospital patient and you know certain drugs or situations may aggravate your RLS, be sure to notify your doctor or the hospital personnel who care for you. If you are not familiar with the drugs they use routinely or you don't know which drugs might cause you a problem, you can get that information on one of many RLS medic alert cards. Several RLS groups have developed professional-looking wallet-sized cards that describe RLS, give warnings about how to deal with someone who has RLS, and list drugs that are likely to trigger RLS symptoms. These cards can be located by doing an Internet search for "RLS medic alert cards." You can also obtain a pamphlet called "RLS and Surgery" from the Restless Legs Syndrome Foundation or their website.

Review your list of aggravators

Constantly maintain your list of aggravators. If your RLS symptoms flare, you can quickly review your list and determine whether something you did triggered the situation. Seeing chocolate listed as an aggravator might remind you of the candy you just ate at a party and explain the sudden increase in RLS symptoms.

Step 6: Reduce Situations

(Prioritize needs)

I F YOU HAVE followed the first five steps of the Reduction Plan, you may have already turned your *beast of RLS* into an *RLS bully*. You may have targeted treatable symptoms, treated coexisting ailments, learned to avoid aggravators, and addressed deficiencies. Despite all these reductions and the resulting improvements, some situations may still be more RLS-provoking than others.

It takes time to reduce all the appropriate variables and to learn sufficient tricks for fighting Restless Legs Syndrome. If drugs are used, it takes time to find the right dosages and combinations. Concentration and distraction techniques take time to develop and practice. It may be a while before you can reduce your RLS symptoms in all at-rest activities. Meanwhile, you need to feel you are in control as soon as possible, and you need to give your body time to rest and catch up.

Prioritize activities

One way to quickly feel more in control is to avoid optional situations where RLS symptoms are likely to appear. Make a list of all the situations where you can almost count on RLS symptoms occurring, then decide which situations are critical to your life and which situations can be avoided, at least for a while.

You may spend your first months, or years, learning to get through high priority activities like getting to sleep or sitting through meetings at work. Later, when your priority activities are very manageable, you can begin working on optional activities, such as leisure reading, watching TV, and taking long driving trips.

Adjust unavoidable RLS situations

If you can't avoid RLS-provoking situations, make adjustments that will give you advantages and help you avoid the worst scenarios. Obviously, you cannot give up the idea of going to sleep. Instead, become familiar with suggestions for good sleep hygiene and give yourself every advantage when trying to sleep. Later in this book, there is a chapter that gives tips for developing better sleep habits.

If you have to see a movie in a theater, try seeing it earlier in the day. Going to a matinee will usually mean the theater will be less crowded and you will be less likely to get trapped in a small space with nowhere to stretch your legs. If you go on a long car trip, try to be the driver. If you have to read a book, read it early in the day, when RLS attacks are less likely. If you have to take an airplane trip, leave early in the day, reserve aisle seats, and follow a well thought-out plan, as described later in a chapter about traveling with RLS.

Recruit support and understanding

Once you have made some progress in reducing the frequency and severity of your RLS in priority situations, you can try to improve some of the optional situations. Meanwhile, explain your plan to your loved ones, so they can support your attempts to avoid potentially horrible RLS situations. When I started consciously working on my RLS survival, I explained to my family that I would not be sitting down and watching television with them in the evenings. If I wanted to watch a show, I sat at the computer and multitasked while the show was on, or I would jump up during every commercial, stretch my legs, and remind myself I was not trapped or restricted to sitting. I often kept busywork handy, whether it was knitting, laundry to fold, or suckers to work over. For a long period, there was no snuggling on the couch during evening television time. It helped a great deal when those around me understood I needed to avoid certain situations while I built confidence and developed my ability to deal with RLS symptoms.

Decide when to tackle a new situation

In this section of your file system, list activities or situations you need to avoid. Begin gathering ideas and keeping detailed notes on ways you might learn to make these situations more bearable. After working on getting to sleep, I worked on going to the movies. Then I worked on being a passenger in a car. I am still working on watching television at night. I have made some improvements, but sitting in a small room watching television when I am tired is still one of my most RLS-provoking activities.

Final Reductions

From beast to bully

WE WOULD ALL like to completely eliminate Restless Legs Syndrome (RLS) symptoms. Realistically, we can expect the Reduction Plan to help us reduce the severity and frequency of our symptoms. By following the six steps of the Reduction Plan, we should be able to turn the out-of-control *beast of RLS* into a manageable *RLS bully*.

An out-of-control case of RLS may not respond well to treatments, but a reduced case of RLS symptoms should respond nicely and cause less interference with your at-rest activities. Your RLS may still be an obnoxious, nerdy bully, but at least you will feel empowered, rather than victimized by it. Beasts can get you, but we can handle obnoxious bullies.

Repeat, repeat, repeat

Revisit the various steps of the Reduction Plan as often as possible. In time, you will add information and need to change some of the information and notes you previously collected.

1. **Reduce PANIC:** New information is showing up every year. Sometimes it seems as if things have slowed down and no new information is forthcoming. Then, when you least expect it, there is a major breakthrough. Never stop researching and learning.

2. **Reduce CHAOS:** As you make changes, your RLS symptoms and behavior will also change. Hopefully, they will become less frequent and less severe. Keep analyzing your RLS behavior and adjusting your treatments and responses. As you reduce the chaotic nature of your symptoms, your treatments may become more effective.

3. **Reduce SYMPTOMS:** As time goes on, you may develop new symptoms that need to be diagnosed and differentiated from your RLS symptoms. Avoid the mistake of attributing all new or increased symptoms to RLS. They may be due to another ailment that is aggravating the RLS.

4. **Reduce DEFICIENCIES:** You may be low on iron one year, but need to reduce your iron supplements the next. The addition of a new prescription heart medication might create a deficiency you never had to address in the past. Continually question whether deficiencies are present and can be alleviated with the use of supplements.

5. **Reduce AGGRAVATORS:** You never know what new medication, food, or activity will suddenly increase your RLS symptoms. Keep on the lookout for new aggravators. If your RLS suddenly gets worse, ask yourself what recent changes might be responsible. Before assuming a medication has lost its effectiveness, ask whether something is temporarily aggravating your RLS.

6. **Reduce SITUATIONS:** As your lifestyle changes, you may find new situations that are prone to produce RLS attacks. Try to avoid these situations until you have time to analyze them and develop a plan for reducing the variables that make your RLS worse.

What is next?

Once you have reduced the *beast of RLS*, you must confront the resulting *RLS bully*. You could do this by going to a doctor and asking for a prescription medication. The doctor and the medication should be more effective at relieving your RLS, once you have it down to bully size. Nevertheless, instead of relying on one pill to fight the *RLS bully*, it is better to develop a comprehensive approach, where several tricks work together. The total approach I suggest is Part II of the RLS Rebel Program, the Bag of Tricks Approach (BOTA).

RLS REBEL PROGRAM

Part II: The Bag of Tricks Approach

Understanding the BOTA

WHEN I STARTED consciously fighting back against Restless Legs Syndrome (RLS), I collected many potentially effective tricks. A large black bag became my RLS trick caddy and was with me whenever I attempted an RLS-provoking at-rest activity. I was never sure which trick I would need, so I took them all. It was a very large bag because I was determined to take control.

I remember priding myself on getting through a six-hour drive to Albuquerque, even though I had to go through my entire Bag of Tricks (BOT) five times and still had to stop to take walks. I shocked myself when I managed to sit through three hours of *Titanic*, even though I was constantly rummaging through my bag, using every trick several times. Feeling I was making real progress, I shared my success stories with others in an RLS email support group. Their response was interesting.

No easy route

Many RLSers told me they had already tried all my tricks, with no success. Others claimed it was too much trouble to go through all those tricks just to find one that worked. Many of them insisted they would rather go the "easy route" and just take a pill.

Before long, we discovered it wasn't so easy to just take a pill. Though pharmaceutical treatments provided some relief, persistent RLS symptoms often needed attention before it was time for the next dose of medicine. We heard reports that some medicines made people's RLS worse or created side effects that were less desirable than the RLS symptoms. Some RLSers talked of having to take "drug holidays" because they had developed a tolerance to a certain drug, rendering it ineffective. The RLSers usually said the medicines were helpful enough to be worth the trouble, but were not the easy way to go.

I knew my idea of always carrying a huge BOT was too complicated and cumbersome to catch on as the best way to fight RLS. Still, we had to have a variety of options. Recognizing the elusive and shifty nature of RLS, I decided we needed a generic plan that stressed a combination of tricks, a systematic approach, flexibility, and the importance of each RLSer customizing a personal program.

It's an approach

My original plan amounted to randomly using all the tricks in my bag. I kept filling my bag with more and more tricks, just to be sure I covered all the bases. I was actually afraid of not having enough tricks with me. I soon realized it was not a question of how many tricks I used, but of whether I had a plan to use them effectively. It was not enough to randomly pull tricks from my bag.

I needed a program in which I could pre-select groups of the most appropriate tricks and use them in a systematic approach. The core of the approach needed to be an attitude of *zero tolerance*. If my first attempts failed, I needed a sure-fire plan to stop an escalating RLS attack so I could get back to my at-rest activity and make it through the activity with my planned tricks. I had to have a way to replace my panic and frustration with confidence and success.

Most of all, I wanted an approach I could teach to other RLSers. How could we gather all the treatment options, pick the right ones for each situation, apply them effectively, and still be ready in the event of failure? In answer to these needs, I developed the Bag of Tricks Approach (BOTA).

Four steps of the BOTA

The BOTA is a guideline all RLSers can use, regardless of what tricks they prefer. The four steps in the BOTA should be followed in order, although they will not all be necessary for every at-rest activity. The first two steps of the BOTA relate to the initials BOT (Bag of Tricks). In Step 1: Gather Your Tricks, the RLSer records information on any RLS tricks that seem interesting and possibly worth a try. In Step 2: Pack Your Bags, the RLSer matches tricks with the activities where the tricks will be most effective.

The last two steps of the BOTA (Step 3 and Step 4), are the Approach (the A in BOTA). In Step 3: Plan of Attack, the RLSer develops and applies a strategy for getting through an at-rest activity, despite RLS attacks that might occur. In Step 4: Relief Plans, the RLSer does whatever is necessary to quickly stop persistent RLS symptoms, even if it means temporarily stopping the at-rest activity. After successfully applying the Relief Plan and stopping all RLS symptoms, the RLSer returns to Step 3: Plan of Attack, applies the best strategies for success, and tries to resume the current activity, using the original Plan of Attack strategies.

The BOTA file system

Using the titles of the four steps of the BOTA you can set up four sections in your file system.

Step 1: Gather Your Tricks

Step 2: Pack Your Bags

Step 3: Plan of Attack

Step 4: Relief Plans

Within the BOTA sections of your file system, you can store information on your RLS tricks and design your approaches for using them. Make these sections work for you. They are your personal RLS workshop space.

Step 1: Gather Your Tricks

(List all treatment options)

Why not one trick?

TRICKS IS THE term I use for all preventative measures and defensive responses to Restless Legs Syndrome (RLS) symptoms. In an earlier chapter, "Rebel Terminology," I explained that the various therapies and treatments we use for RLS remind me of magic tricks; sometimes they work and sometimes they don't. When they do work, they often give the illusion of having cured our RLS, when they've only brought us temporary relief.

Many people have high hopes of finding one simple, inexpensive, and safe treatment. Some people come close, finding a treatment that takes away most of their RLS symptoms most of the time, but in many of these cases, there are trade-offs. One therapy may stop the RLS, but give you insomnia. Another may make you sleepy, but not stop the RLS. Some tricks work, but are too cumbersome to have with you when needed. Other tricks are noisy and disturb others. There does not seem to be one simple answer.

The following are four reasons for using a Bag of Tricks (BOT) rather than relying on one trick to do it all:

1. Every trick has its purpose. If you are chasing more than one complaint, you may need more than one trick. Some tricks address RLS urges, while others are meant to dis-

tract you, induce sleep, or relax muscles. You wouldn't use a sleeping pill to help you sit still through an afternoon meeting, and you wouldn't use a bag of popcorn to distract you while trying to get to sleep.

2. No single trick is 100 percent reliable in all RLS situations. A normally reliable trick might become ineffective if you unknowingly added an aggravator to the mix (e.g., ate chocolate, had too much caffeine, took an antihistamine). Even if one trick usually worked, the added aggravator might call for extra tricks.

3. Unforeseen circumstances can make you glad you do not rely on one trick. What if you ran out of your usual trick? What if you left on vacation and forgot your medications? Would you have to forgo a movie if you got to the theater and realized you didn't have money for popcorn (to distract you), forgot to bring your suckers, or didn't pack your therapy band (for stretching)? What if you got on an airplane and realized you had forgotten to reserve an aisle seat? If your airplane were detained or you were held over in an airport for the night, would you panic if your best tricks were in the luggage that was already checked through?

4. Special situations might forbid the use of your favorite trick. What if your favorite tricks were not allowed, or were unusable? Would you be okay if you had to discontinue all RLS medications before going into surgery? What if your best trick was to walk, but the airplane was in turbulence and the *Fasten Seat Belts* sign was on? What if you couldn't walk, due to surgery, an accident, or a stroke?

These are just a few reasons for never settling on only one trick. Always have several tricks ready to use, and continue gathering ideas for new tricks to try, in case your current tricks fail or are unavailable.

Two types of tricks

There are two types of RLS tricks: *no-prop tricks* and *prop tricks*. No-prop tricks are always the best, because you "can't leave home without them" and they don't cost a cent. No-prop tricks include *zero tolerance, bully noise*, distraction, anger, walking, stretching, and self-massage. Some of these take time to learn and perfect, but once you learn them, you will always have them ready to use.

Prop tricks include prescription drugs, herbal remedies, vitamins, and supplements. They also include things like hot baths, hot tub soaks, computer games, herbal teas, suckers, certain clothing (tight stockings, elastic wrap bandages), aroma therapy (candles, oils, sprays), massagers, vibrating heat cushions, bicycle pedalers, foot cushions or steppers (used to increase circulation by simulating walking motions), magnets (strap-on, insoles, mattress pads), and many more. Of course, there's always the great trick of sexual activity, but I never know for sure if that counts as a prop trick or a no-prop trick. I just know it's distracting enough to stop an RLS attack. Later chapters will discuss these tricks and how to effectively use them.

Three warnings about tricks

There are three warnings you should heed when choosing your tricks. The first is to guard your pocketbook. RLS tricks can be expensive. When you are frustrated, sleep deprived, and feeling victimized, it is easy to justify spending any amount, as long as it helps. The problem comes when the new expensive trick does not help or you find there was a cheaper way to do the trick.

When I first heard of percussive (pounding) massagers, I quickly bought one for $200. It was expensive, but worth it to me to have something that would pound my legs. However, I soon found a practically identical product, under a different name, for $60. I actually did a side-by-side blindfolded comparison (I like to tell people I used two blindfolds, so it was a 'double-blind' study). Much to my dismay, I could tell no difference between the two massagers. I could have purchased the cheaper one and saved $140, and considering I never really got into the habit of using the thing, I wish I had not been in such a hurry to buy the latest miracle product. Be careful of anything that sounds too good to be true, or is too expensive. There is a chapter later in this book on how to decide if something might be worth trying.

The second warning is to be aware of the potential danger of any trick you try. Almost all tricks have the potential to be dangerous. I knew one lady who walked at night to relieve her RLS. Normally, walking would be safe, but she had also taken sleeping pills. She ran into walls, bumped into furniture, and tripped over rugs before falling and spending the rest of a night on the floor in fear and pain.

Prescription drugs come with warnings. Other tricks require you to do your own research, check with your doctor, and take into consideration all your personal variables. If I told you to rub your legs vigorously in response to an RLS attack, but you had a rash, fibromyalgia, or lack of feeling in your legs, my advice might be dangerous. If I told you to use an herbal supplement or over-the-counter medicine and you were already taking a prescription drug that had the same effect, you might get too much of a good thing. If I talked you into using my expensive percussion massager and you had severe osteoporosis, it might be the worst advice you ever received.

You have to be the decision maker and guardian of your own safety. I always tell people, "If something works for you, it's because it is potent. If it is potent, then it is 'potentially' dangerous!" Use all treatments with extreme care and respect.

The third warning is to maintain the effectiveness of each trick by avoiding sole reliance on it. A trick can lose its effectiveness in three ways. First, as in the case with medications, your body can become tolerant to the trick. Second, routine use of only one trick can make you complacent, causing you to implement the trick less efficiently than when you first started using it. Third, your RLS symptoms may have increased for some reason, causing your favorite trick to appear less effective. In fact, it might be as effective as always, but the increased RLS symptoms are more than it can handle. By always using a combination of tricks, we can allow our favorite tricks to do their job, while we are prepared with extra tricks to handle special situations when symptoms escalate.

Keep detailed records

Over the years, you may come across hundreds of tricks to relieve RLS attacks. Obviously, you can't try them all. And if you "try only one new thing at a time," you will be lucky if you can remember all the tricks you want to try. Make notes in this section of every good idea you find. You may not need it right now, but someday, when you are planning a long driving trip or you are suddenly having problems getting to sleep, you will be happy to have a good list of choices to review. You may want to list or record the following three categories of tricks:

1. **Tricks I am currently using.** Be careful to note dosages, describe how the trick is used, and note important information, such as brand names or how often you use the trick. If you use an herbal tea, for instance, include the brand and name of the tea, how many bags you use, what the ingredients are, and how much water is used. If you use a prescription drug, be sure to record the name, dosage, and what other medications you are taking with it. You might also note any side effects and other comments that will help you remember your re-

sults with each medication. This information will be invaluable if you change doctors and need to review what has worked or not worked.

2. **Tricks I have tried that didn't work or stopped working.** You might make a note of why you stopped using certain tricks. Were there side effects? Were there other variables determining the effectiveness of the trick? Is it a trick you might try again someday? If a trick stops working, keep your information about it. You might have reason to try it again when your *beast of RLS* has finally been reduced to *RLS bully* status. A calcium supplement that didn't seem to help in the past may help after your RLS symptoms are reduced to bully size. It will be very helpful to know exactly what you took so you can make adjustments in amounts, brands, or combinations.

3. **Tricks I am interested in trying someday.** People will give you ideas and you will come across articles about new tricks, but you will not always have time to research and try every new trick. Make notes about new ideas in this section of your file system. When you are frustrated with your current tricks, you will be happy to have a list of new ideas to consider.

Step 2: Pack Your Bags

(Match treatments with activities)

Pack selectively

My first Bag of Tricks (BOT) contained most of the tricks I knew for dealing with Restless Legs Syndrome (RLS), even if they were not useful in the activity I was about to do. Since then, I have realized I can be selective. I take only the tricks that work best in the situation at hand.

Decide which of your RLS tricks work best in each situation. For example, sleeping pills or sleep inducing herbal teas might be good to have along if you are staying in a hotel and need to insure a good night of sleep, but a sleeping pill would be the wrong trick to have along if you were trying to sit still and enjoy a movie. Likewise, a sucker would not be a practical trick to take to bed with you.

Plan ahead

Packing selectively means you think ahead and anticipate what tricks will work. By doing this, you will always be prepared, and you will avoid the feeling of panic and frantic frustration that comes when an RLS attack catches you off guard and unprepared. Too often, RLSers rely on sincere hopes of having no RLS. Hopes fade, however, as the inevitable RLS attack occurs, leaving the RLSer playing catch up with a raging set of symptoms. It is nearly impossible to think clearly and act with confidence when you are fighting already out-of-control urges to move.

Many at-rest situations will improve with forethought and special preparation. Learn to make adjustments ahead of time, such as dressing comfortably for long trips or movies, reserving aisle seats, leaving room between yourself and others in an audience, and always making sure you can get out and stand somewhere and stretch without bothering anyone. And of course, remember to carefully pack and take along your BOT.

Pack combinations of no-prop and prop tricks

When you are thinking ahead and planning what tricks might work best in an upcoming RLS-provoking activity, be sure to consider both prop and no-prop tricks. Your no-prop tricks will not be something you actually put in your bag. Instead, they will be something you plan to use if RLS symptoms start. As you look down your list of no-prop tricks, picture how you might use brushing, massage, or walking to relieve symptoms during your upcoming at-rest activity. With a combination of no-prop and prop tricks, you will be ready for any RLS symptoms that occur.

Pack different tricks for different types of RLS

Your choice of tricks may depend upon the type of RLS attack you are experiencing. I have several types of RLS that respond differently to treatments. Sometimes the urge to squirm comes from a feeling like my leg is hollow and someone is running a bottle brush up and down inside it. When the urges are mild to moderate and caught early, they respond well to no-prop tricks (e.g., distraction). They also respond well to the prop trick of stretching with a therapy band.

When I get irresistible urges to move my arms, I can respond with a brushing technique. An overall squirmy panic feeling responds well to walking, exercise, herbal tea, or a hot tub soak. Sometimes, especially when I am watching television, the RLS symptoms begin as squirmy urges in my legs, but eventually they knot my thigh muscles. Knotted thigh muscles require stretching and massaging. Analyze your types of RLS (see the chapter "Reduce Chaos" in the Reduction Plan section). Know when symptoms are likely to occur and pack your BOT accordingly.

Keep a packing list for each activity

When I was first learning about selecting appropriate RLS tricks, I made lists of the most effective tricks to use in each at-rest situation. Before leaving for the movies, a car ride, or an airplane trip, I reviewed my BOT packing list for that activity. With practice, I learned to quickly gather the best tricks for each situation. There are some tricks I always take on an airplane, and if someone suggests a night at the movies, I know just the things I need to grab, on my way out the door. Later, you will find detailed information on various prop and no-prop tricks. You will also find a whole chapter on airplane travel. The following lists will give you an idea of the type of packing lists you might write for yourself before doing certain activities.

Airplane Travel

- Wear my most comfortable clothes (loose pants or shorts, shoes that are easy to remove, and layered tops for ease in adjusting to temperature changes).

- Use airlines that allow reserved seats so I can be sure to have an aisle seat.

- Be the last to board the airplane.

- Take food.

- Take my therapy band, portable CD player, headphones, and busywork.
- Take herbal tea and sweetener in a mug.

Movies or Concerts

- Get popcorn or take peanuts.
- Get an aisle seat.
- Scope out walls or corners where I can stand, if needed.
- Take suckers.
- Wear comfortable clothing.
- Take a therapy band to stretch legs and arms.
- Go early in the afternoon.
- Be well rested.
- Be careful of certain plots (silly comedies) which provoke RLS.

Driving a Car

- Be the driver.
- If I have to be a passenger, try for the front seat.
- Wear comfortable clothing and shoes.
- Take CDs with music or narrated books.
- Take handwork.
- Take suckers.
- Use my heated vibrating seat cushion.
- Plan frequent stops.

Lighten and adjust your BOT

At first, when I tried to use music to get to sleep, it did not work. Later, I was able to get to sleep, but only after listening to the whole CD and picturing myself dancing to the music. Eventually, I would hear the first song and be out cold in minutes. Now I seldom need the earphones and CD. Instead, I just think about the songs and picture my feet dancing. I am usually asleep before I know it. It is nice to not always need my CD player, headphones, CDs, and charger, but there are still times (e.g., long airplane trips) when I make sure they are in my BOT.

At first, you will have a full Bag of Tricks. You will carry extra items, in case none of the tricks work or you are suddenly in an unexpected at-rest situation. Eventually, you will find out which tricks are reliable and which are easiest to have handy. With careful planning, based on experience, your BOT should become smaller. As you perfect your responses to RLS, you will build confidence and make adjustments accordingly. Be patient.

Review, repack, and restock

After an at-rest activity, evaluate your success and prepare for the next time. In other words, review your current list of tricks for the activity, make changes according to the experience you just had, and then repack your BOT. If you are working on your ability to get to sleep at night, wait until morning to do your review. Morning will be the best time to analyze whether you used the best music, wind-down routine, or medicine regime.

As you review your tricks, you may decide a trick is too cumbersome, has undesirable side effects, or is too heavy to carry. If so, take the trick off your BOT packing list for that activity. If you come across a new idea for the activity you just finished, be sure to add it to the list for next time.

If your tricks are consumable (e.g., medicines, herbal teas, suckers), be sure to restock, and if you give away your tricks to other frustrated RLSers, be sure replace the items. I was on a long flight from Tucson to Atlanta when, out of the corner of my eye, I saw someone's leg stretching out in the aisle. It was an RLS-type stretch I have learned to recognize. After talking with the lady and telling her all about RLS, I gave her my therapy band. She used it for the rest of the trip to Atlanta and according to her email, she also used it throughout her return trip. Another RLSer, who received his first therapy band at one of my lectures, forgot to bring it with him when he flew from Florida to California for a Restless Legs Syndrome Foundation national meeting. When I heard how upset he was for not having his trusty trick with him, I gave him one of my extra bands. As soon as I removed it from my BOT, however, I put a reminder note in the bag, "Get another therapy band!"

Step 3: Plan of Attack

(Your plan for getting through an activity)

What if RLS symptoms show up?

IN THE EARLY morning hours of a sleepless night, I was chatting on the computer with an RLSer whose symptoms were driving her crazy. Her medications weren't doing the job, she had long ago given up on any self-help methods, and for the most part, she was out of ideas. I finally convinced her to try a large cup of my favorite Tension Tamer tea, which she had on hand but had never gotten around to trying. Between the tea and the mental distraction of our chat, her Restless Legs Syndrome (RLS) symptoms finally subsided.

When I suggested she go to bed and get some sleep, her response was, "I'm afraid to go to bed. What if the RLS symptoms show up?"

My response was, "You can be sure they will show up. Count on it!"

She was shocked by my comment and I was shocked by her fear. I suddenly realized she had no idea what she would do if her RLS symptoms started. The minute the slightest RLS feeling occurred, she figured the battle was lost. With no strategy to fight back, she felt extremely vulnerable. Apparently, the only way she could get to sleep was if she were totally free of RLS symptoms.

A whole new concept

Many RLSers fear the appearance of their RLS. They see no way to continue an at-rest activity once RLS symptoms begin. When every attempt to sleep has been thwarted by RLS attacks, the RLSer often prefers staying wake to the thought of going to bed and facing another round of RLS symptoms.

Instead of feeling defenseless and fearing the occurrence of RLS symptoms, RLSers need to ask, "What precautions can I take to prevent symptoms from occurring?"

More importantly, they need to ask, "If I fail to prevent the symptoms, how will I respond when they appear?"

For an RLSer who is used to having RLS symptoms continually disrupt normal activities, it will be a totally new concept to finish the activity even though RLS symptoms are present.

Develop a two-stage Plan of Attack

The first part of your Plan of Attack is the *preparation stage*. As you approach an at-rest activity, you can take precautions, make adjustments, and eliminate many RLS-provoking variables. Preparation efforts can actually lead to an RLS-free experience.

The second part of your Plan of Attack is the *attack stage*. Though you prepare for the activity with every intention of thwarting RLS symptoms, you must approach the activity with the idea that residual symptoms are waiting to ambush you. You may need to attack RLS symptoms before they attack you. Just assume they will be there and start your best tricks when you start your activity.

The *preparation stage*

As you approach the start of an RLS-provoking activity, take steps to minimize the likelihood or severity of RLS. What aggravators can you avoid? What situations can you adjust? What tricks can you apply, even before starting the activity?

1. Avoid a huge meal before going to a movie, concert, or getting on an airplane.

2. Plan to see the movie matinee, when RLS is less likely to occur and theaters are less crowded.

3. Avoid going to your seat until the last minute (e.g., on airplanes, in movie theaters).

4. Plan airplane and car travel for early in the day.

5. Wear comfortable clothing (e.g., loose styles, layers, shoes that can easily be removed).

6. Reserve aisle seats on airplanes and in theaters.

7. Consider seats in back rows or near side walls so you can stand and stretch.

8. Avoid aggravators (e.g., antihistamines, red wine, other alcoholic drinks).

9. When approaching bedtime, practice a well defined wind-down routine.

10. Take medications that need time to start working.

With no preparation, you are more likely to have severe RLS attacks. By taking time to prepare for the activity, you can minimize the severity and sometimes entirely prevent the occurrence of RLS symptoms. In this section of your file system, record things you can do in advance to decrease the chance of RLS symptoms occurring during your at-rest activity.

The *attack stage*

You do not want to be caught off guard and unprepared when RLS symptoms appear. If you are unprepared, the tendency will be to struggle to remain still. The risk is that you will slip into complete RLS panic or have to abruptly stop the activity and chalk it up to another ruined experience, thanks to RLS. The best idea, of course, is to have an attack plan, where you know exactly what tricks to use and how to make them most effective.

It is common for RLSers to feel trapped and anxious when they are totally unprepared for escalating RLS symptoms. One day, I found myself in that type of situation when I was on what should have been a relaxing two-hour car ride with my husband. About a half hour into the trip, I went from happy and relaxed to being full of panic and tension. My RLS had kicked in with a vengeance. I had completely forgotten to bring along any tricks, so I tried to be still and just endure the symptoms.

I thought to myself, "Just sit still. They will stop."

Instead, they got worse. I knew I was in trouble when I found myself staring at the door handle and imagining opening the door and escaping from the car, even though it was going 75 mph. That is how powerfully and dangerously RLS symptoms can attack if you are unprepared. Luckily, we arrived at a rest area just in time for me to bolt from the car and walk, walk, walk.

My experience is so much better when I am prepared for RLS attacks and get a head start using my tricks. On a car trip, I try to bring busywork, snacks, or music to distract me. If I am overly tired, I try to take a nap. At the first feeling of an urge to wiggle, I quickly and purposefully adjust my position, stretch my legs, clear the area around my feet, and maybe organize a few things, as a way to distract myself and feel in control of my environment. I might take off my shoes.

I also might say to the driver, "Hey, I'm getting some RLS symptoms. Please keep an eye out for a place to pull off safely. If I am not successful at fighting off these symptoms relatively soon, we may have to stop."

It helps to know someone is looking for my escape route and I am not as trapped as I might feel.

When symptoms appear, never settle for just hoping they will disappear on their own, and never assume you must immediately stop your at-rest activity. There are ways to overpower RLS symptoms and proceed with the activity. In this section of your file system, you can record strategies and tricks you find effective in helping you get through at-rest activities.

Ammunition for your attack stage

My best plans for attacking RLS use a combination of prop and no-prop tricks. I may try no-prop tricks, like simulating walking movements or trying to start a stimulating and distracting conversation. In addition, I may try prop tricks, such as suckers, handwork, herbal tea, or calling someone on my cell phone. Some attack plans are a series of tricks, meant to be used in a specific order. Later in the book, I will share my personal Bag of Tricks Approach (BOTA) for getting to sleep. I will describe how the four tricks in the attack stage of my Plan of Attack are designed to work in a very specific order. In some at-rest activities, the order of the tricks is irrelevant, as long as the individual tricks can be used quickly, aggressively, and confidently.

Start your attack early

Some activities and situations are so likely to provoke RLS, it makes sense to start your attack before the symptoms show up. If you wait for symptoms to establish themselves, you may become too restless and frustrated to put up an effective defense. It is always easier to apply your tricks early and get a head start toward relieving symptoms.

The best example of this is the activity of getting to sleep. Just as a football team would start its offensive strategy in the locker room, RLSers should start their offense in the *preparation stage*. Go to bed with every variable already adjusted in your favor. Then start your attack as soon as you get into bed. Do not wait for symptoms to start. That way, you will be less tired and have clearer thoughts than if you struggled with RLS symptoms for a while before starting your attack. If the urge to wiggle never shows up, you have won. If it does show up, at least you will be ahead of the game and already on a roll toward relieving symptoms.

Don't let RLS disable you

RLS is recognized by the American Disabilities Act (ADA) because it substantially limits a major life activity (sleeping). The ADA protects against having disabilities that deprive us of doing our jobs and enjoying normal public activities. For many people, RLS has become a disability and causes them to give up important activities. Sleep deprivation and the inability to sit still have forced many RLSers to quit their jobs. RLS symptoms can easily turn a usually competent and healthy person into a disabled victim. Some people try to keep RLS from disabling them by pretending it is not a problem. They head into at-rest activities with no preparation and no plan for responding to symptoms. Their only plan is to tough it out or hope RLS symptoms will not appear. This is a setup for disaster.

Pretending RLS does not have the power to disable you is not the way to prevent it from affecting your activities. I do not like to consider myself disabled any more than active wheelchair-bound people like to think of themselves as disabled. Nevertheless, it is important for me to recognize the potential for RLS symptoms to disable and disrupt if I do not plan ahead and have my strategies ready to deploy. People in wheelchairs learn to think ahead, inquire about wheelchair accessibility, and surmount problems presented by doors, stairs, or narrow passages. Just as wheelchair-bound people must check for entrances and exits with ramps, RLSers need to look for places to stand and stretch when the RLS symptoms become severe. We must pack appropriate tricks and carefully prepare for an activity so it will be enjoyable and bearable. We must make our at-rest activities achievable by always using an effective Plan of Attack.

Step 4: Relief Plans

(Your plan to stop symptoms, immediately)

I WISH OUR PLAN of Attacks were guaranteed to work. Wouldn't it be nice if we could count on being able to sit through a movie by just eating popcorn or briskly massaging our legs? What if we could always get right to sleep by listening to music and doing a few stretches? It would be so nice if we could do our Plan of Attack and expect to consistently enjoy long car rides and airplane trips.

Sadly, those scenarios are not our realities. A skillfully developed and executed Plan of Attack will usually subdue mild to moderate Restless Legs Syndrome (RLS) symptoms and allow us to continue our at-rest activity. There will be times, however, when RLS symptoms will persist and rage out of control. We must be willing to interrupt the activity and quickly shift our focus to stopping the RLS symptoms. We can't effectively continue with our Plan of Attack when our RLS symptoms are taking over. The purpose of the Relief Plan is to stop the escalating symptoms. Once they are stopped, you can return to Step 3: Plan of Attack and try to complete your at-rest activity.

Understand the difference in Plan of Attack and Relief Plan

The Plan of Attack focuses on completing an at-rest activity. The Relief Plan puts a stop to RLS symptoms that are more than your Plan of Attack tricks can control. Let's take a look at the difference in a Plan of Attack and a Relief Plan in the same at-rest activity.

> **Plan of Attack at a movie theater:** Prepare yourself for a good experience by wearing comfortable clothes and arranging to see a matinee. Get to the theater early, making sure you get an aisle seat. Buy a big bag of popcorn to keep distracted. As you watch the movie, shift positions periodically. If RLS symptoms begin, briskly rub the area where they appear. Press your feet to the ground alternately, as if you were walking. If the symptoms get worse, temporarily interrupt the at-rest part of the activity (sitting) and move straight to your Relief Plan.

> **Relief Plan at a movie theater:** Do what it takes to immediately stop the RLS symptoms. Stand along a side wall or go to the back of the theater. Do heel lifts or calf stretches. Quietly march in place. If symptoms are still bothering you, take a walk to the bathroom or go to the lobby and get a drink of water.

In this scenario, the Plan of Attack should help you stay seated and enjoy the movie. The Relief Plan helps you put an immediate stop to persistent RLS symptoms. Once symptoms are stopped, you can take your seat and reapply your Plan of Attack tricks.

Do Relief Plans always require you to stop the activity?

In most cases, the Relief Plan requires you to temporarily stop your at-rest activity. One exception is seen in the example of the movie theater. The first attempts at the Relief Plan suggested that the person merely stand by a wall or in the back of the theater and do heel lifts. While doing this, the person could still be watching the movie. The at-rest part would be interrupted, but the activity could continue.

Another example of continuing an activity while applying a Relief Plan might occur on an airplane. A later chapter, "Traveler's RLS," explains how RLSers can apply Relief Plans when they are required to remain in their seats. In most cases, however, the activity will be stopped when you apply your Relief Plan. For example, if you can't get to sleep with your Plan of Attack, you will have to get out of bed, do the Relief Plan, and then resume the activity of getting to sleep.

Practice *zero tolerance*

As long as symptoms remain mild and intermittent, you can apply your Plan of Attack tricks and continue the activity. Sometimes the distraction of applying the tricks is enough to make the RLS symptoms disappear. If the symptoms escalate, however, it is extremely important to use *zero tolerance.* Never stay put and allow RLS symptoms to gain momentum and escalate out of control. Stop them immediately by applying a reliable Relief Plan.

It is not easy to know when to go from trying to deal with mild symptoms (your Plan of Attack) to quickly applying *zero tolerance* (a Relief Plan). While you are focusing on applying your Plan of Attack, be on the lookout for escalating symptoms.

The minute you see them heading out of control, tell yourself, "This is not working. The squirmy feelings are getting worse by the minute! I've got to stop them, right now!"

The most important trick you have is one that helps you enforce *zero tolerance.* When you plan ahead for an RLS-provoking activity, be sure you have at least one great Relief Plan trick in mind that will help stop symptoms immediately. Even if you have to keep walking, be confident you have a way to stop RLS symptoms and keep them under control.

Alternate between Step 3 and Step 4

Be prepared to continually alternate between Step 3: Plan of Attack and Step 4: Relief Plans. Once you have applied your Relief Plan and stopped the RLS symptoms, go back to Step 3, resume your activity, and reapply your Plan of Attack. If RLS symptoms escalate again, quickly move to another Relief Plan.

When you are first learning to use the Bag of Tricks Approach (BOTA) you may spend more time doing Relief Plans than your Plan of Attack. Later, after many adjustments and a great deal of practice, you will find your Plan of Attack will work more reliably and most of your time will be spent enjoying your at-rest activity.

When I first learned to use the BOTA, I'd constantly alternate between my Plan of Attack and my Relief Plan. The Relief Plan always worked, in that it successfully stopped my RLS symptoms. But when I would get back in bed, the RLS symptoms would return too powerfully for my unskilled abilities at using my Plan of Attack. After months of working with this program, I was tired of having to repeatedly get out of bed to apply the Relief Plan.

I said to myself, "I know what is going to happen. I will get out of bed, stop the symptoms, and then be right back here, trying my Plan of Attack again. Just this once, maybe I will allow myself to stay in bed and try my Plan of Attack one more time."

To my amazement, my tricks worked and I fell asleep. It took a long time and a lot of practice to get to that point, but most of all, it took confidence and determination. Do not give up. Just when you think something will never work, it will surprise you and make all your efforts worthwhile.

Develop several Relief Plans

Relief Plans should be designed in varying levels of length and effectiveness. If you have one failed attempt to get to sleep, it would not make sense to spend an hour doing a long Relief Plan. Instead, try a short and easy Relief Plan, such as walking to the kitchen, getting a drink of water, and doing a few quick stretches. Then get right back to bed and try your Plan of Attack again. If your next attempt fails, you can try a Relief Plan with a more complex set of tricks.

In the Relief Plans section of your file system, you will want to list tricks that are the most reliable for stopping RLS attacks. It would help to list them in order, beginning with the ones that are fastest and easiest to apply and ending with those that take more time and more effort to apply. As you alternate between Step 3 and Step 4 of the BOTA, work down your list, choosing Relief Plan tricks that are progressively more complex. The following is an example of progressive levels of Relief Plans you could use in conjunction with trying to get to sleep at night. The various levels of Relief Plans are separated by attempts to get to sleep. If your Plan of Attack does not get you to sleep within approximately fifteen minutes, move on to the next Relief Plan.

> **Plan of Attack (10:00–10:15 P.M.):** Use your best Plan of Attack for getting to sleep. If it fails, do a quick Relief Plan.
>
> **First Relief Plan (10:15–10:20 P.M.):** Use the slight distraction of walking to the kitchen, getting a drink, stretching, and going to the bathroom. Go right back to bed.
>
> **Plan of Attack (10:20–10:35 P.M.):** Apply your Plan of Attack for getting to sleep.
>
> **Second Relief Plan (10:35–10:55 P.M.):** Make a strong cup of herbal relaxation tea and sip it while playing computer games. Some people use teas or supplements with chamomile, kava kava, or valerian to induce sleepiness. If you use an *as needed* medication, it might be a good time to take it. As soon as your legs calm down (hopefully, within fifteen to twenty minutes) go right back to bed.

Plan of Attack (10:55–11:10 P.M.): Apply your Plan of Attack for getting to sleep.

Third Relief Plan (11:10–11:40 P.M.): Try mental distractions, such as paying bills, organizing, or cleaning. Look for RLS aggravators, such as indigestion, pain from another ailment, or stress over upcoming events, and try to treat those issues. Stay up for about thirty minutes or until you are sure the RLS symptoms have subsided and your body is calm. Then go back to bed.

Plan of Attack (11:40–11:55 P.M.): Carefully apply your Plan of Attack for getting to sleep.

Fourth Relief Plan (11:55 p.m.–12:30 A.M.): Take a long, hot soak in a hot tub, bath, or shower.

Plan of Attack (12:30–12:45 A.M.): Apply your Plan of Attack for getting to sleep.

As you can see from the times in this example, you could alternate five Plan of Attacks and four Relief Plans in approximately three hours. It may seem like it is taking all night, but it really is not. In fact, you would have time to repeat the process before 4:00 A.M. (the hour when many RLSers find they can finally relax and get to sleep, even on their worst nights).

Is the BOTA a ridiculous waste of time?

If it seems silly getting in and out of bed doing Relief Plans, just think of the alternative. You could stay in bed, thrashing, turning, and wiggling, until you are so frustrated you want to scream, or you could spend the entire night pacing the floor and dealing with out-of-control RLS symptoms. By alternately using your Plan of Attacks and Relief Plans, you confidently and consistently stop RLS symptoms and practice your strategies. You may not get to sleep, but you are definitely not wasting your time.

Not-so-popular Relief Plans

Some Relief Plans are for emergency situations, when nothing else works. Sometimes we have to put aside our goal of completing an at-rest activity while we make it our highest priority to stop all RLS symptoms. Other times, we have to make drastic changes in the activity just so we can finish doing what we set out to do. The following are examples of Relief Plans that get the job done of stopping RLS, but they may not be the most popular alternatives.

1. **Sleepless nights Relief Plans:** There are times when you just have to get some sleep. One of my tricks for these nights is to move to the guest room and sleep alone. Sometimes it is easier to get to sleep when I know I can wiggle without disturbing my husband. I can thrash, toss, turn, growl, whine, and hit the pillow. A little adrenaline rush is always good for calming RLS symptoms. I have been tempted to use this Relief Plan more often, but I really do not want "sleeping in the guest room" to be the solution to my problems.

2. **Audience restlessness Relief Plans:** If your RLS symptoms are unusually strong and persistent, you may have to give up on accomplishing your activity. For one reason or another, there are times when nothing you do will help you be still. At times like that, if you are not enjoying the movie or concert anyhow, focus on doing whatever you need to do to stop RLS symptoms. You might as well be comfortable. Of course, if it is a mandatory meeting, you may just have to get creative and persevere.

3. **Travel Relief Plans:** If you are taking a car trip, one of your Relief Plans will probably be to stop for a short walk and stretch. If that does not work and you are not on a set schedule, try changing your plans. Stop for

lunch, take in a museum, or a stroll through a park. Do something to get totally distracted from being in the car. If you are in an airplane, you may have to spend a good deal of time out of your seat. Explain your situation to the flight attendants and work within the rules. On a long trip overseas, I spent quite a bit of time standing in the extra wide exit row behind my chair. I leaned over the back of the chair and watched the movie on the monitor in the back of the seat in front of mine. All the time, I was doing little marching steps to keep moving.

These are not ideal Relief Plans, but there are times when they are necessary. We must always know we can stop the attacks, safely, even if the methods are not the most popular.

Focus on successes

Remember, every time you apply a Relief Plan, you are stopping your RLS attacks. In the past, you might have endured excruciating RLS symptoms and been frustrated and worried about not being able to stop the sensations. Now, each time you successfully use a Relief Plan, you will be gaining control and confidence, which will greatly improve your efforts to survive with RLS.

Look for small successes. Needing one less Relief Plan means success. Staying until the end of the movie, even if you had to stand by the wall, can mean success, especially if you kept the RLS symptoms from escalating. Getting to your destination on time without needing multiple walking stops can mean success.

Success will also be seen in your attitude. In the past, you might have walked the floors all night, thinking, "How will I ever stop these awful feelings? Here goes another sleepless night."

Now, you will notice yourself focusing on your next Relief Plan. You will feel confident, knowing you can quickly stop your RLS symptoms and have another good shot at getting to sleep.

Focus on all the times you are able to stop RLS symptoms. Notice the times when your Plan of Attack works and you get through at-rest activities that previously were unbearable. Your patience and persistence will bring you success.

YOUR BAG OF TRICKS

Understanding Your BOT

IN EARLIER CHAPTERS, I introduced the Bag of Tricks Approach (BOTA), as a way of gathering a variety of tricks and using them to prevent and respond to RLS attacks. This section gives more detailed suggestions for developing and utilizing your unique BOT.

The next chapter, "No-Prop Tricks," reviews tricks that do not need packing, because no special item is needed for the trick. Two valuable no-prop tricks, concentration and music, are covered in separate chapters. Both of these tricks require special understanding and skill in order to use them effectively. Music can also be considered a prop trick if devices are used (e.g., CD player, headphones).

The final three chapters of this section discuss prop tricks. The chapter "Prop Tricks" will discuss useful items that can be packed in your BOT. Possibly the most desired and perplexing prop trick, prescription medication, is discussed in a separate chapter. The final chapter of this section gives tips on how to decide when a treatment idea is too good to be true or is worth your time, money, and effort.

Does this mean I always have to carry a BOT?

Anytime you fortify yourself with several useful tricks for dealing with Restless Legs Syndrome (RLS), you are technically using a BOT. However, carrying an actual Bag of Tricks is not always necessary. You might find you can pick up prop tricks along the way (e.g., popcorn, crossword puzzles). You can eliminate the need to carry an actual BOT if you perfect the skill of using no-prop tricks (e.g., walking, concentration, massage).

When I first started using the RLS Rebel Program, I carried a large duffle bag on airplane trips. On car trips, I carried my tricks in a small canvas tote. At home, I stashed tricks in a basket by my TV chair. In my bedroom, I kept a collection of tricks available on my nightstand. At first, I had more tricks than I needed, but I wanted to be sure I was never caught without something that would work when RLS attacks occurred. My BOT became smaller as I learned what tricks were most reliable, and I carried even less when I became adept at using no-prop tricks.

Consider variety, purpose, and timing

Discussions about RLS will often include the statement, "What works for one person, may not work for another." We also hear people say, "What worked for me this time, might not work next time." Because this is true, we must think in terms of variety, purpose, and timing.

1. **VARIETY:** A variety of choices will be available if you consider prop and no-prop tricks when you pack your BOT. If you use prescription medications, you might consider having a variety of types. In one situation you might need a sleep medication, but in another you might need something to just help you keep calm. If you rely on daily medications, you might also want to have emergency medications to be used on an *as needed* basis. Also be sure to have reliable alternative or self-help tricks to fill the gaps when medicines do not work or when your legs are restless before it is time for your next dose.

2. **PURPOSE:** In previous chapters, I discussed the two steps that are part of the *approach* for using your BOT.

The purpose of the Plan of Attack is to get through an activity. The purpose of the Relief Plan is to stop an RLS attack quickly when your Plan of Attack fails. While packing your BOT, think of the purpose of your tricks. What tricks will be good for your Plan of Attack and what tricks will work best for your Relief Plan?

Ask yourself, "What will I need for getting through the activity?" Then ask yourself, "What will I need if that fails and I have to start a Relief Plan to stop the escalating RLS symptoms?"

3. **TIMING:** By observing your RLS tendencies, you might notice times when your RLS tends to be the worst and times when the very same activity will not produce a single urge to move. It could be that your outbound flight goes very smoothly, but your return flight produces miserable RLS. You might get through the first half of a concert with no problem, but after the intermission, your legs go crazy. We need to be careful to not become complacent just because we make it through a typical RLS situation with no problem. The next time might not be as easy. This topic is covered in greater detail in the chapter "Traveler's RLS."

Your BOT contents will constantly change

The contents of your BOT will constantly change. The BOT you take to the movie theater will have different items than the bag you take on an airplane trip. You will continually analyze the usefulness of various tricks and weed out those that are not worth having along. You may change your CD selections as you discover which music works best. Medicines will change. You will find new and different gadgets. You will need fewer props as you perfect your ability to focus on mental distractions and use other useful no-prop tricks.

Keep your BOT handy

It would be a good idea, especially when you are first developing your BOTA, to have one place where you keep most of your RLS tricks. If you store several sizes of tote bags with your tricks, you can easily grab the best bag for the tricks you plan to use. If you have to spend time rounding up the tricks or finding something to carry them in, you are less likely to take your BOT.

Keep a list of tricks in the same location as your BOT. You will not always have time to contemplate what tricks you might need. If you have your listed items grouped according to activity, it will be easy to grab what you need before sitting down to a movie or starting a long car ride. It is also helpful to list no-prop tricks so you have a visual reminder that you can walk, massage, or use concentration.

As with the whole RLS Rebel Program, you will need to customize your BOT to your needs. If it is quick to assemble, easy to grab, and simple to replenish, you are most likely to make good use of it.

No-Prop Tricks

AN *ACTUAL* B**AG** of Tricks (BOT) is the bag of visible props you keep on hand to deal with Restless Legs Syndrome (RLS). A *virtual* BOT is an invisible group of tricks that do not use props, but can be effective in preventing and responding to RLS. Some no-prop tricks are easy to learn and take little practice to apply effectively. They are more of an attitude and a quick response (e.g., the concept of *zero tolerance*, distraction, walking). Other no-prop tricks are fine-tuned skills that take time and practice before they can be successfully applied (e.g., concentration, brushing, *bully noise)*.

There are many advantages to perfecting the use of no-prop tricks. You do not have to remember to bring them with you, they weigh nothing, and they do not take up room in your BOT. If you develop a useful virtual bag of no-prop tricks, you will never be unprepared or caught off guard by a raging RLS attack, and best of all, no-prop tricks cost nothing.

Use *zero tolerance*

When I was editing the manuscript for this book, I got to this point and read a comment I had already made (more than once) and would probably repeat several more times before the end of the book.

I almost deleted it, but then I said to myself, "Jill, if you kept writing it, you must really believe it. Leave it in."

So here goes, one more time: If I could give only one suggestion for surviving with RLS (everybody sing along now) I would tell you to use *zero tolerance*. When you use *zero tolerance,* you aren't just ignoring symptoms and hoping they will go away. Instead, the instant you become aware of RLS symptoms, you are responding with your best Plan of Attack or Relief Plan tricks.

If you feel RLS urges start while you are watching television, you can apply *zero tolerance* by quickly rubbing your legs. If you are in an airplane when the urges start, you can begin a simulated walking motion. If you are trying to get to sleep, you can quickly put on your headphones and listen to music. The important thing will be your readiness, speed, and determination to stop the RLS attacks immediately.

The longer you allow RLS symptoms to develop, the more severe they will become, and the harder they will be to stop. *Zero tolerance* will give you a better chance of staying put and finishing your at-rest activity. If your quick efforts fail, you will have to immediately stop the RLS urges by using some sure-fire tricks from your Relief Plan. Your quick decision to move to your Relief Plan is another way to show you will not tolerate RLS urges.

Zero tolerance can also work as a kind of behavior modification approach. When you train yourself to repeatedly have a quick response to RLS symptoms, your body and mind eventually learn to expect quick relief. You will be training your body and mind to react quickly and successfully. With any luck, the *RLS bully* will realize it is not worth pestering you. Previous responses of anxiety and panic will give way to behaviors based on feelings of empowerment and confidence.

Here is an example of how *zero tolerance* can lead to behavior modification. Picture a mother talking on the phone while her children play impatiently at her feet. The children, wanting Mom's attention, start nagging and acting rowdy. If

Mom ignores them, they will continue to raise their voices and pester each other. This is the same as if you were trying to ignore RLS. It will just get worse as it tries to get your attention.

The mother's best move is to tell the person on the phone, "I will call you right back."

She should hang up the phone, deal strictly with the children, and then place the call again. If the children act up again, she should repeat the process, hanging up the phone, dealing with them, perhaps in a more unpleasant and unrewarding way, and then place the call again. By responding to the children's unfavorable behavior quickly and consistently, the mother is using *zero tolerance*. Once the children realize their mother is not helplessly tied to the phone but is ready to immediately and strictly deal with their behavior, they will think twice about acting up while she is on the phone.

If the mother consistently follows this plan, putting down the phone and dealing with the children, they will no longer see mom's telephone time as permission to misbehave. Likewise, *zero tolerance* will teach you and the *RLS bully* that you are not fair game just because you decide to sit down or go to sleep. You are not tied to your seat or glued to the bed. You can move quickly, and you can stop the bully in its tracks.

Think of walking as a blessing

Many RLSers think walking is a bad thing. They complain, "I was up, walking the floors, all night." In many ways, walking is a blessing, not a curse. Imagine if you could not walk off an RLS attack. Walking should be viewed as one of your most reliable and effective no-prop tricks.

Walking is most effective if it can be done with a purpose, rather than aimlessly pacing around the house. Tidy up the house, climb the stairs a few times, do some dances or stepping routines. Try repetitions of jumping jacks or calf stretches while leaning into a wall. Movement that is routine, rhythmic, or purposeful, will work as well or better than walking, but remember that walking is fine all by itself.

Simulate walking

There are times when walking would be helpful, but is not possible. For instance, if you are in the center of a row at a theater production or in a middle seat on an airplane and the *Fasten Seat Belt* sign is on, walking might not be an option. In these cases, you can simulate walking without getting up. You can buy special two-chambered pillows or mini-stepping machines, which help simulate walking while you are still seated (see "Prop Tricks: Non-prescription"). However, you can do the same motions without the devices, making the movements a very effective no-prop trick.

To simulate walking without using props, place both feet flat on the floor. Press down with one foot, while barely touching the floor with the second foot. Next, press down with the second foot and lighten the pressure with the first foot. Your thighs should feel the motion, as if you were walking. Your concentration and the exercise itself can be very useful for fighting off RLS symptoms. Imagine yourself walking down a road. If you stop your imaginary walk and the RLS returns, just start your simulated walking again.

Stretching exercises

There are times when you need movement, but walking is not enough. Certain types of RLS attacks may cause your calf or thigh muscles to harden, tighten, or cramp. If this happens, it might help to do some stretching exercises. One good exercise for RLSers is heel lifts. To do these, stand up, lightly hold on to something for support, and then raise up on your toes, bringing your heels as high off the ground as you can. Some folks repeat these rhythmically until they have done hundreds of them. Another good stretch is to stand on a step, with just the front part of your foot on the step, letting your heels hang lower than the step. Be careful to always do slow, steady stretches, rather than bouncing.

Use massage and brushing

Another no-prop trick that helps you respond immediately with *zero tolerance* is to massage or brush the area that feels like squirming. There are professionals who specialize in massage and brushing therapies, but you can successfully perform your own simplified renditions of both of these activities. Whether you rub your muscles or someone else provides the massage, it can quickly stop RLS symptoms and relieve tightening muscles.

The professional practice of brushing can be very complicated, using a special brush and following a strict set of guidelines. The technique is used by physical therapists in treating people with sensory disorders. Brushing is also used as a therapy for autism, as well as a self-help technique for people believing it provides healing. After reading several long lists of instructions on how to correctly use brushing therapy, I modified the idea to my own RLS needs.

My way of brushing is very simple. I pretend I have imaginary *RLS rubbing cream* in my hand, and I apply it wherever I feel the urge to wiggle, whether it be in my calves, my thighs, my feet, or my arms. If the sensations move, I quickly chase them with the imaginary cream as if I am snuffing out fires. The object is to squelch the feelings before they spread. I know this sounds silly, but it almost always works. The only time it fails is when I wait too long to try it and the symptoms are already too severe. I try to start brushing the minute I feel an RLS symptom.

I believe the success of brushing lies in using several no-prop tricks at once. The friction of brisk rubbing causes a soothing sensation of heat. At the same time, I become distracted by the "shushing" sound of the fast movements. As I am spreading the imaginary cream, I am concentrating on where the feelings are appearing, and finally, my brushing creates movement, and we know movement will stop RLS symptoms. Therefore, brushing employs the no-prop tricks of distraction, concentration, and movement.

The trick of brushing is perfect for RLSers who have symptoms in their arms. If you have RLS in your legs, you can relieve the sensations by walking. It is pretty difficult to relieve symptoms in your arms, just by walking. Brushing your arms can thwart RLS symptoms before they escalate into a serious problem.

When I fail to act quickly, my irresistible urges to squirm can lead to knotted thigh muscles. When that happens, brushing is not enough. Instead, I switch to a deeper and firmer massage technique. I like to use the base of my hand to rub deeply and slowly over the washboard-like muscles. A rolling pin works the same way, but it is a prop trick and is not always handy. My hand works just as well, making it a perfect no-prop trick.

If you are fortunate to have an RLS *angel* offer to give you a massage, be sure to develop good communication and give your special person useful feedback. I have heard many RLSers say their partners tried to help by providing massages but did it too hard, too fast, or not in the right area. You must communicate. Do not expect another person to know the best way to massage away your RLS symptoms. Explain and experiment until the two of you become an effective team against RLS. Remember, the person providing the massage wants you to feel good. Help that person be successful by offering feedback as to what works.

Practice the skillful art of *bully noise*

Imagine that RLS symptoms are a result of useless signals being sent to your limbs, saying, "Move, move, move! Do not sit still!"

Since we can't just ignore those nagging signals, we must overpower them or drown them out with something louder and more persistent. We must generate what I call *bully noise*. The term *bully noise* came to me as I thought of how similar this concept is to a scene you might see on a school playground when one child is being bullied by another.

The bully might taunt the victim with, "Na, na, na, na, na! You can't sit there. You're in my spot. Come on, move, move, move!"

The badgered child will instinctually put fingers in ears as a first attempt to shut out and ignore the bully, but just as RLSers eventually realize they can't ignore obnoxious urges to wiggle, the tormented child on the playground realizes that fingers in the ears do not totally block out the bully's taunts. What can the poor child do? With fingers still in the ears, the child could start yelling loudly. It doesn't matter what is being yelled, as long as it's louder than the bully's nagging.

Just yelling, "Na, na, na, na, na . . . laddie da, da . . . I can't hear you!" is enough.

This is how *bully noise* works with RLS, too. During an RLS attack, it is as if the brain is sending useless bully taunts to the legs and arms. If I can concentrate extremely hard on something else, making louder brain noise than the useless noises urging me to wiggle, then I will not be bothered by the bully signals. This is definitely not an easy concept to implement. It took me months to master the skill of using *bully noise*, but once it was learned, it became easier to apply and has continued to work like a charm.

To drown out the useless signals with *bully noise*, you can do something as easy as getting into an argument or heated discussion, working math problems, reciting a poem, or re-membering lyrics to a song. When I learned that I could create *bully noise* with distractions, I told my husband I was going to need his help. I told him that if he saw me *ootching and scrootching*, he had my permission to distract me and get me thinking about something else. It was his free chance to start an argument, but the understanding had to be that I would always win.

Many types of environmental noises can act as *bully noise*. You may have heard of people using white noise to drown out street noise. An air conditioner in a hotel room can drown out the sounds of cars going by. If you concentrate on the sound of an air conditioner, a motor, or a ticking clock, the sound may be enough to overpower the bully signals to wiggle.

Take fast deep breaths

There are many relaxation programs that start you out taking slow, deep, cleansing breaths, and then guide you to slowly relax from the tip of your toes to your head. I don't know about you, but with me, by the time I take one slow, relaxing breath, my RLS symptoms will have me wanting to jump off the bed. Slow and relaxing is practically an oxymoron to RLS. And yet, I highly recommend taking breaths to relax, as long as they are quick, deep breaths.

Sometimes, I swear I hold my breath while waiting to go to sleep. Taking fast, deep breaths will put an immediate stop to that silliness and prevent any tendency to be tense or anxious. The catch to using deep breathing to fight RLS is to take fast, deep, and exhausting breaths. I quickly take in as much air as I can, as fast as I can, and then I let it out as if someone just punched me in the stomach and knocked the wind out of me. A couple of those breaths and I feel as though I just ran a race and collapsed at the finish line.

After long-term successful use of my Plan of Attack, it is easy to become complacent and overlook some very important steps. When an unusually difficult RLS night suddenly occurs and I just can't seem to get to sleep, I find it is always good to go back to taking those two very deep breaths. The breaths seem to send a signal to my mind and body that I am finally ready to give up and stay in that spot for a long time. I can't be holding back any tension or fear of being still when I have just exhausted myself with those two deep breaths.

Consider sex

I wonder how many syndromes or diseases would have sex recommended as a useful therapy. It may be the only good thing about RLS. Of course, any suggestion to consider sex comes with the warning that it be appropriate to your age and lifestyle, and be totally safe. In most cases, sexual play will stop RLS attacks, at least for a while. In many cases, it will stop it for the remainder of the current at-rest activity. There could be many reasons for this. First, it is movement, and we know movement will stop RLS. Second, it can be rhythmic, and we know rhythm or routine movements are useful as mental distractions. Third, it usually involves heavy breathing, which is effective in reducing tension and relaxing us. Fourth, it creates a heart-pumping rush of adrenaline. All of these points, and more, make sexual play an excellent no-prop trick. Of course, some people would argue that sex is actually a prop trick.

Distraction

When our first child was beginning to toddle around the house and get into things, my husband and I were determined to teach him the meaning of "No!" We thought one good "No" should make the baby stop the unacceptable behavior and automatically change to a new and acceptable behavior.

We ignored all the great advice of our parents, who said, "Just move him away and give him something to distract him."

Not our child! He was going to learn the meaning and appropriate response to "No!"

Almost 30 years later, I am preaching to my children, who now have babies of their own, "Try to distract them. There will be plenty of time to explain what 'No' means later."

The same can be said of dealing with RLS. You can sit in one place and stubbornly try to gain control, or you can quickly distract the *beast of RLS* and get him to leave you alone. Distraction can come in the form of a heated argument, working a crossword puzzle, listening to music, or organizing your briefcase or purse. In the following chapter, I will give detailed suggestions for using concentration as a form of distraction. You can train yourself to create a reliable distraction by focusing on predetermined thoughts that will create effective *bully noise*.

My favorite distraction is music. When I learned to use music, it was a prop trick involving CDs, a player, and headphones. I would concentrate on the music until my brain was so distracted, it couldn't hear the sounds of the *RLS bully*. Eventually, I learned to create the distraction by just thinking about the music. I could imagine the song and imagine myself clogging (dancing) to it. Before I knew it, I had turned music into the perfect no-prop trick. Following the next chapter, "Concentration," there is a chapter with specific tips for using music as a reliable RLS trick.

Concentration

I wish I could tell you to ignore your Restless Legs Syndrome (RLS) symptoms and just relax, but I know it's not possible. If you just turn away from the urges or try to ignore them, it will create a mental void, which the *RLS bully* seems to love. The trick is to fill that void by concentrating on something. When you focus on something intently, you will no longer be aware of the ongoing RLS urges to wiggle.

Have you ever sat in a restaurant and been unable to focus on the conversation with the person across from you because you were so distracted by a loud conversation at another table? Have you ever tried to talk to someone while that person was distracted by a football game or television drama? We all have difficulties focusing when something louder, more persistent, or more exciting is begging for our attention. It is as if we need ear plugs and mental blinders. Wouldn't mental blinders be great? Picture the blinders they use on horses so they can't see to the side. What if we had mental blinders that could keep our brains focused and prevent our ability to think of any undesirable or distracting urges to wiggle?

When you use the trick of concentration, it is as if you are putting on mental blinders as you focus your attention on whatever you have chosen. The nagging urges of RLS will still be there, but with practice, you will become skilled at focusing all your attention on the subject of your concentration.

It takes a considerable amount of practice and skill to use concentration as an RLS trick and to use it well enough to overpower the temptation to pay attention to RLS symptoms.

RLSers have told me, "Concentration doesn't work. I tried it once, but the RLS symptoms were too strong."

When I hear this, I know that person does not understand how much work and practice goes into effectively using the trick of concentration. If your first attempts fail, you must continually refine your technique, train your body to respond, and improve your ability to stay focused.

Prepare your mind

In order to concentrate successfully and end up either sitting still or going to sleep despite an ongoing RLS attack, your mind must be prepared to accept the intended result. Even though you say you would love to get to sleep, your thoughts may be telling you to expect a night of restlessness, walking, and frustration. Therefore, if you are using music or visualization as a concentration tool to induce sleep, you will have to be sure you are open to the idea of actually getting to sleep and enjoying a peaceful night.

For an RLSer, bedtime is often a time of frustration, disappointment, and failure. After years of facing RLS problems when trying to sleep, you may have unknowingly conditioned yourself with suggestions or repetitive thoughts that say you do not enjoy your bed, you do not look forward to bedtime, and you do not expect to feel rested in the morning. With these negative thoughts and expectations, you will be working against any attempts to get a good night of sleep, because your mind will be prepared for the worst outcome, rather than for the best results. If this is true for you, you will have to consciously change your thoughts about yourself and how you relate to sleep. RLSers need to see sleep as something we can do, will do, and look forward to doing.

Ask yourself if you believe you can get to sleep tonight. You do not want to think of yourself as a non-sleeper. You must visualize yourself as a solid and successful sleeper.

Avoid making negative comments like, "I don't sleep at night."

Be aware that if you keep saying, "I can never get to sleep until about 4:00 A.M.," that will become the routine your body will expect to keep.

Avoid pessimistic thoughts like, "I sure hope RLS doesn't keep me awake again tonight."

Instead, be realistic about the chances of RLS showing up, but maintain positive thoughts like, "When RLS shows up tonight, I will be ready to take control and get right to sleep, despite the obnoxious urges to move."

As you get ready for bed, practice positive mantras, such as:

"I can't wait to get to bed."

"I will fall asleep quickly and easily."

"I will sleep until the alarm goes off in the morning."

"I have all my tricks ready, and my Plan of Attack is reliable and ready to use."

Carefully choose your focus

When you use concentration, you will be focusing on something other than the intended result. Do not focus on sitting still or sleeping. You should not be thinking about whether you are tired, how your legs feel, or how trapped you are in the middle of the row at a theater. Instead, concentrate on music, counting sheep, imagining a marching band going by, or counting how many times an actress makes a certain gesture. The subject of your concentration must be something you can clearly and easily hear, see, or visualize.

We know that movement is helpful in stopping an RLS attack. Try visualizing your body in motion (e.g., walking, running, dancing, bicycling). Experiment with which visual holds your attention best.

It is easiest to imagine things your body and mind are familiar doing. If you have never done aerobic exercises, it would be hard to visualize yourself doing them. On the other hand, if you walk the same path around your neighborhood three times a week, you could probably visualize every house along the way and every turn in the road. You might be able to visualize yourself kicking a stone as you walk down the street. If you have a hobby that has several intricate steps, you may be able to picture every step or motion of that hobby. One RLSer told me he could visualize himself refinishing a piece of furniture, step by step.

When I imagine my dance routines, I *feel* every step as I think about it. If I tried to imagine downhill skiing, I could not create a useful visual from that. All my body remembers about skiing is the sheer terror of skiing uncontrollably downhill (straight for a tree) and ending face-first in the snow. I'm afraid that would bring on a nightmare, rather than restful sleep.

Discipline yourself to stay focused

I cannot stress enough the importance of investing plenty of time in becoming a skillful user of concentration. To be successful, you must force your mind to stay on one chosen subject. This takes a great deal of discipline. Most people are used to letting their thoughts freely jump to whatever is demanding the most attention. If you are trying to get to sleep using concentration, it is common to have your thoughts flip to focusing on the RLS symptoms, listening to sounds in the house, or thinking about plans for tomorrow.

If your thoughts wander, quickly yank them back to focusing on the music or visuals you have chosen for your concentration. It is best to go back to the beginning of your visual or the start of your music each time your thoughts wander.

Learn to recognize the moment you lose focus, and say to yourself, "Oops! I'm off track. Go back to the beginning and try it again."

If you continue from where your mind wandered, it will not work. Remember, this is a skill and you are developing the ability to *stay* focused. It is not a matter of getting through the visual or song. Getting through it is not what makes it work. The goal is to increase the length of time when you are so focused nothing (especially RLS symptoms) can distract your mind.

When I first tried concentrating on one of my clogging routines, I could not get beyond the third step of the dance without my mind wandering. It took many nights of focusing, concentrating, and starting the routine from the beginning before I was able to concentrate enough to run through the whole routine in my head. Eventually, I mastered the art, and I would fall asleep before the routine was finished. I was amazed at the amount of discipline and effort it took to keep my mind on dancing and to actively picture every aspect of it.

Believe it will work

There is a saying (often used in relation to jumping horses) that you should throw your heart over the fence and the rest (you and the horse) will follow. When you use concentration to get through an at-rest activity, you need to throw your heart and expectations into the desired goal. See yourself sleeping or envision yourself staying seated until the end of the trip. You cannot be sitting there wondering if you can do it or wondering if concentration will work. With 100 percent of your focus on concentrating, you must believe that you will succeed in your at-rest activity.

If you focus on sleeping, it will actually work against you. It is like the saying, "A watched pot never boils," but in this case, "A watched RLSer never falls asleep."

Merely ask yourself, "Am I ready to go to sleep now?"

If the answer is yes, start concentrating on your music or whatever technique you use, having faith and confidence your plan will work. It may seem like all that brain activity would keep you awake, but it won't. Sleep will come, even though your mind is busy focusing. When I am effectively concentrating, I am not aware of RLS urges, nor am I aware of sleep approaching. It just happens.

When I was first getting good at using concentration, I would actually play games with myself, trying to get to the end of a CD or to the end of visualizing a dance routine before falling asleep. It took me a while to realize the more adept I became at using the skill of concentration, the faster I would fall asleep and the less chance I would have of ever hearing the end of the CD. In fact, sometimes I was asleep before the end of the first song.

Your ability to believe in your concentration skills can be sabotaged by negative thoughts you may not be aware you are thinking. If you find yourself afraid to go back to bed (for fear of RLS symptoms showing up) it could be a sign that you do not believe in your ability to concentrate and get to sleep.

You can't possibly be confident in your abilities if you are thinking, "I'll never be able to get to sleep, tonight."

You must believe you can use your concentration skills to get to sleep, even if RLS attacks occur.

Consider these tips

As you practice your concentration skills, consider some of the following tips that I have found useful in improving my own abilities to use concentration.

1. *Get comfortable.* It is hard to concentrate when you are thinking about how warm you are, how cramped you are, or how hard the mattress is. Wiggle and squirm until you are comfortable with your space. Dress for comfort and make sure your surroundings are conducive to the length of time you hope to be sitting or sleeping.

2. *Take deep breaths.* After you achieve a comfortable position, try taking a few fast, deep breaths in and out. They should be quick, frustrated, relinquishing breaths of exasperation. These breaths will be a fast way of releasing the tension in your body and will allow you to sink into the bed or sit back and relax in your TV chair. If your mind wanders or you begin to panic, take a couple more deep breaths, just in case the first ones have worn off. I am often amazed at how tense I am and how much that tension prevents me from sleeping or sitting still. A couple of fast, deep breaths can become your way of telling your body you are ready to be still.

3. *Use key words and comments.* When you phrase questions or statements to help you get to sleep, your choice of words can emphasize your commitment and determination.

   You might say to yourself, "I am ready to fall asleep now and to stay in a deep sleep until morning."

   Using the word *now* is a way of telling yourself this is to be immediate — not ten minutes from now, but *right now*. If there is any reason you can't fall asleep *now*, you should get out of bed, take care of whatever is on your mind, and then start your Plan of Attack again. Committing to the word *now* is a signal of your readiness.

   The word *deep* and the phrase *until morning*, require you to think about not only getting to sleep, but about the quality and length of your sleep. Using the word *fall* suggests that you are not holding onto anything, but drifting into another state of being. We tend to say we just want to *get* to sleep, but in reality, we want to go much deeper into the sleep state and stay there until morning.

Most people react to RLS attacks with thoughts that express panic, fear, or disappointment. Instead, we should react with thoughts of being in control and staying relaxed.

At times, I have been successful saying to myself, "Just relax. You are not going anywhere. Nothing is going to hurt you."

Sometimes, especially when the RLS is just beginning, these comforting words actually work to calm the urges to wiggle.

One RLSer told me he had decided to take control by growling at his RLS. When symptoms started, he let out a big, "Grrrrrrrrrr!"

He said it worked beautifully, even though it scared his two dogs and sent them running for cover.

4. *Choose a good subject.* When I was in labor with my first child, I was told to get through the pains by focusing on something in the hospital room. The sign on the bathroom door said, "For Patients Only." If I stared at the *F*, the labor pains felt sharp, like the edges of the *F*, but if I stared at the *O*, everything seemed rounded and soothing.

Believe it or not, if you stare at the wrong object, listen to the wrong music, or think the wrong thoughts, it can make the RLS urges worse. The slightest variable can make a difference. Soft, slow, flowing music will make my RLS worse. Fast, lively, loud music works much better. Find something that allows your mind to focus—and then focus, focus, focus.

5. *Consciously focus.* No matter how familiar you are with your music or visualization, you have to concentrate on

what you are hearing, visualizing, or staring at. If you are too familiar with the music, the tendency is to use it as background music and allow your mind to wander. If you are not familiar enough with the path or activity you are visualizing, your mind will wander. Focusing is what is important. You can lay there passively listening to music for thirty minutes, but unless you focus on it and think about what you are hearing, it will not work as a concentration trick.

6. *Create useful visualizations.* As you are finding things to visualize and focus on, consider creating an imaginary treatment for your RLS symptoms. In Step 2 of the Reduction Plan (Reduce Chaos), I suggested you analyze your RLS symptoms and behaviors.

I made the comment, "If you can describe it, you can predict it. If you can predict it, you can treat it."

If you can imagine or visualize the RLS sensations, you can develop customized visuals of treatments to match the sensations. For instance, if you have the sensation of ants crawling in your legs, you might visualize a little Tasmanian Devil running around, scarfing up all the ants. Mmm . . . yum! If you envision your RLS as electrical sensations shorting out connections in your legs, you might imagine repairing the wiring in your legs, or you might just imagine yourself pulling the plug and stopping the sensations altogether. If you envision itchy irritations, you might visualize a smooth, creamy liquid coating the inside of your legs.

The important thing is to take your time and keep experimenting until you visualize a soothing treatment that matches your visualized symptoms. Because I see my RLS as a bottle brush scratching the inside of my legs, I have tried picturing the bristles on the brush being filed away or softened, until they provide a nice, soothing massage. To be honest, this is not a technique I ever mastered, but I can see its potential. It makes sense that if you spend so much time visualizing how strange and irritating the feelings are, you need to spend an equal amount of time imagining them subsiding under treatment.

7. *Develop the skill.* You may be thinking, "This is all too much work."

    There is no doubt that it takes a lot of work to become skillful at using concentration, but once you get good at it, it will work quickly and effortlessly. This kind of concentration is a skill that must be developed. Think of how long it takes and how much effort a young child puts into learning to balance and ride a bike. Balancing on two tires seems like an impossible skill to learn at first. But eventually, it is no trouble at all. When you are faced with the choice of walking the halls in frustration for hours or listening to your music and forcing yourself to concentrate for a few minutes, the choice will be obvious.

8. *Stick with it.* When you are first learning this technique, you may find yourself listening to all the songs on an album and thinking you are not getting to sleep. Do not give up too soon. You may be dropping off to sleep without realizing it. It is like being in an elevator and stopping at each floor. Each song takes you a little closer to your destination of sleep.

    It will definitely work against you if you are lying there thinking, "But I'm still awake! This isn't working."

    Sometimes it is not until the album is over and you are lying there with no sound remaining that you will finally enter a deep sleep.

9. *Count your blessings.* Sometimes when I feel the RLS symptoms begin, I am filled with resentment.

   I am sure we all suffer from moments of thinking, "Why me? Why can't I just relax like other people?"

   One night, when I was recovering from surgery, I whined to my husband, "I am so sick and tired of this darned RLS every night. I just want it gone!"

   Calmly, he asked, "What will help?"

   I suckered right into it, answering, "Putting on the earphones and listening to my music."

   He said, "Maybe you should try that."

   Even when I have a reliable remedy for RLS, I may still resent the fact I need to use it. In order to make the decision to use a trick like concentration, I must stop feeling sorry for myself, and start taking control of my current situation.

   Though I may feel too tired and resentful to try, I have to remind myself, "The alternative is not good. Either I expend the energy to listen to the music or I'll be walking around, or on the computer for the next two hours, paying for it with exhaustion the next day."

   When I hear myself ask, "Why me?" I try to follow with, "Why not me?"

   At least I have a plan to follow and an approach that will keep me sane. And, after all, I *can* get up and walk. That is still a blessing to be counted.

10. *Anticipate the learning curve.* I have heard people say, "Oh, I tried concentration, but it didn't work for me."

    This never surprises me. There is a learning curve or a period of time when you are still practicing the technique and learning to make it work for you. There are many variables to work out, like changing from earphones to a pillow speaker, trying different kinds of music, finding new and different things to focus on, and figuring out ways to prepare yourself for the best results. It took me several months before I could get to sleep by relying on music or concentrating on a visualization. At first, I would listen to a whole CD and not be asleep, or I would have to keep getting up and doing my Relief Plans. A time finally came when I could fall asleep after a few songs, and then after only one song. These days, I am often asleep before the first song is over. Part of this learning curve is because you are training your mind and body to respond to concentration.

At first, it may not work at all, but eventually, you will learn to stay focused and will find yourself asking the question, "Should I get out of bed, start my Relief Plan, and just stop these crazy feelings, or should I try concentrating one more time and see if I can get to sleep?"

The day will come when you try concentration one more time and it will work perfectly. More importantly, it will work faster. It may take a whole CD to get you to sleep when you are first learning this technique, but eventually you will learn to fall asleep during the first song or two.

11. *Use the power of suggestion.* At first, it will take considerable time and effort to achieve a mental state where you can effectively concentrate, but eventually, you will need only the suggestion of concentration (e.g., the start of a song, the beginning of a visualization, a few lines of a poem).

Years ago, my husband learned self-hypnosis. When he was just learning the process, he spent twenty to thirty minutes relaxing and trying to reach the desired state of consciousness.

Eventually, he was able to reach a state of total relaxation by merely saying to himself, "The moon is blue."

Periodically, he found it helpful to refresh his skills and practice the entire relaxation process from the start.

Do not be discouraged if you are spending a considerable amount of time learning to concentrate effectively. Once the process is learned and you repeatedly achieve the desired result of being able to be still and finish your at-rest activity, the process will become faster and easier to use. In fact, you may find that it takes only a few seconds and a short phrase to put you in a state of mind where you are totally unaware of your RLS urges.

12. *Use it or lose it.* If you do not use your concentration techniques for a while, you might find your skills get rusty. On a suddenly awful night, you may try your old trick of concentration and find it doesn't work nearly as well as you remembered. Perhaps you forgot some of the important steps or you lost your skillful ability to stay focused. It is actually easier to use concentration if you have nightly bouts of RLS and can make it a routine practice. Using concentration as part of your nightly ritual, whether RLS is present or not, will help you avoid losing your focusing skills.

13. *Write it down.* Once you have developed your best strategies, write them down. Make note of every variable and thought that makes concentration work for you. If it's been a while since you have used your concentration skills, your notes will help refresh your technique.

14. *Respond consistently to wake ups.* If you wake up during the night and have to get out of bed to relieve your RLS symptoms, use your concentration skills to get back to sleep. The same skills that got you to sleep when you first went to bed should work just as well during the night.

15. ***Do not expect 100 percent success.*** Concentration works for me about 90–95 percent of the time. The times when it doesn't work are when I get an overall body restlessness that sends me into a sheer panic or when something is aggravating my RLS. If I have caffeine too late in the day or have excessively stressful thoughts, concentration will not work. Sometimes, concentration fails if I start too late and the RLS attack is already out of control. Once a sense of panic sets in, I usually cannot regain my focus without using my Relief Plan to quiet things down.

   I used to have a couple days each month when the trigger of my hormonal cycle seemed to overpower my ability to use concentration. That is when I would resort to hot tea and computer games while waiting for my body to settle down. Then it was a matter of going back to bed and trying to get to sleep before the RLS urges returned and became too strong. On very rare occasions, it still ended up as another sleepless night.

16. ***Use concentration for many at-rest activities.*** Concentration is a trick that can be used for almost any activity where RLS shows up. Of course, if you were driving a car, you would not want to put yourself into a trance or subconscious state. But you can safely focus on things that keep you alert (e.g., the cars around you, your driving skills, songs on the radio, talking out loud). When watching a movie, you might be able to do apparently silly things like counting the number of times someone smiles or critiquing the makeup or costumes.

17. ***Read for details.*** Relaxing with a good book or reading a newspaper can be one of the most difficult activities for RLSers. For many years, as soon as I tried reading the newspaper, my RLS would begin and panic would set in. Reading a TV guide, catalogue, or magazine would also bring on horrible RLS urges. My tendency was to re-

spond to the urges by immediately reading faster, barely getting any information, and finally giving up and putting the paper down. Actually, it was more like *throwing* the paper down and fleeing, as if I'd been sitting on an anthill.

I believe now that the quick reading made things worse, because it created too many little bits of information at once. For some reason, when RLS strikes, attention to detail and engrossment in one subject seems to help the most. I had to learn to slow down, focus, and concentrate on smaller chunks of input. Now, when I feel the sensations start while I am trying to read, I force myself to choose an article, read it thoroughly, concentrate on the descriptions, and imagine every scene in detail. It sometimes helps to read out loud, one word at a time, exaggerating the pronunciation of each word. Before long, I relax and can read the rest calmly.

Of course, as with everything related to RLS, efforts to read for details will not always work. There will be times when the only option is to stop trying to read, move around until the RLS urges subside, and then try the reading activity again.

18. *Start early.* Expect RLS every night when you go to bed. It should not be a shock when it shows up. Start your concentration tactics early. Prevention is the best policy, but if an RLS attack begins, early intervention is critical. Never allow the urges to escalate and send you into a full blown panic.

    To use concentration as a response trick, rather than as routine prevention, you must become quick to recognize the start of RLS symptoms.

    It has to be a matter of thinking, "My RLS is acting up. I have to start concentrating right now."

    If you hesitate and tell yourself, "My RLS is acting up. I'll keep an eye on it and see if I have to do something about it," it may escalate too quickly and thwart your ability to use concentration.

19. *If it fails, move on to your Relief Plans.* Set yourself up for success by learning to use concentration on relatively mild RLS attacks. If concentration fails to work, move right to your first Relief Plan and stop the symptoms quickly. Get up, do chores, walk, or do whatever it takes to settle the RLS as quickly as possible. Do not try to be a hero and suffer through it. Once you get it calmed down, resume your activity and quickly apply your concentration methods, even if you think the RLS symptoms are gone for good. It is always better to be safe than sorry.

Using Music and Other Audio

THIS CHAPTER WILL focus on tips for using various audio sources as tools for concentration. Most of the references involve using music, but other audio sources can be equally useful. In fact, you may find you prefer using audio books, white noise machines, or subliminal programs. As you read about examples of using music, feel free to substitute examples of other types of audio.

No-prop or prop?

This chapter has been strategically placed between the chapters on no-prop tricks and prop tricks. When you are first learning and practicing the skill of concentration, it is much easier to listen to music or audio books than to come up with your own thoughts, tunes, or visuals in your head. You will need props, such as headphones, CD players, or pillow speakers. After you are disciplined to concentrate, you might be able to free yourself from the props and just imagine the sounds in your head. Music is something you can imagine or hear in your head, making it a potentially wonderful no-prop trick.

When I first learned to listen to music as a way of getting to sleep each night, I became totally dependant on my props. I had to have my speaker pillow, my portable CD player, and my special CD. I relied on this method so much that if I were on a trip, I would have to take all my music props with me. I would replace the hotel pillow with my sound pillow, search for a plug near the bed, and have to remember to grab it all when I checked out of the hotel. The thought of being without all my props was frightening. At the time, they were one of my only treatments for Restless Legs Syndrome (RLS). I would not dare be away from home without them.

Eventually, I learned to concentrate on the tunes and dance routines in my head and was able to get to sleep without needing physical props. There are still times, however, when I use all the musical props. After surgery, I used my earphones and music while I was still in the Intensive Care Unit. I take my audio props when I am on airplanes or long car trips. When my husband and I take motorcycle trips, I have music piped into speakers in my helmet. The music helps me to sit still and avoid RLS problems during the ride. I just have to hope the beautiful scenery and excitement of the ride keep the music from putting me to sleep.

Consider direct input

If you want to practice concentration using audio input, consider the advantages of using headphones or a pillow speaker. By having the speakers close to your ears, you will be using what I call *direct input*. If your audio is coming from speakers on the other side of the room, you may be distracted by other room sounds. With direct input, it is easier to stay focused.

It is also easier to focus on certain tasks when the sound comes from direct input. There are times when I try to spend time in my kitchen, cooking, doing dishes, or cleaning up a mess. No sooner do I get there than I think of something else to do (e.g., email, phone calls, changing the TV channel). If I put on my radio headset and have music piped directly into my ears, I can stay on task and finish what I need to do in the kitchen. It is as if it demands my attention and shuts out thoughts that normally would make me wander from the task at hand.

If this process sounds familiar, it's because it is another example of *bully noise*. The sounds going straight into your ears can actually demand more of your attention than the RLS urges to wiggle or squirm. Using direct input can make the difference of whether you can successfully use music or other audio sources to overwhelm the RLS signals to move.

Consider portability

For several years, I used a portable CD player for my *concentration* music. These days, I use my MP3 player. It's smaller, it does not require CDs, and it can easily be loaded with new music or audio books. Laptops and DVD players are other options for listening and concentrating. Regardless of what you use, try getting something small, durable, battery efficient, and able to run off AC power. You do not want to end up with dead batteries and a machine that will not work when you need it the most.

Be sure your player has a shut-off feature that is automatic and silent. You do not want to have to wake up in order to turn off the machine, and you do not want to be awakened by a loud click when it shuts off. At first, I used a tape player that worked very well until it reached the end of the tape and shut off with a loud *click* that defeated all my hard work of getting to sleep.

Carefully choose headphones

Headphones come in many varieties and prices. If you can, try them on in the store. Some go into your ear, while others go over your ear. I cannot wear the type that is supposed to push into the ear and stay there. They fall right out of my ears. If I want to lay back and sleep with headphones on, I can't have ones that go around the back of the neck. Here is a list of things to consider when it comes to headphones.

1. Are they comfortable, with no pressure, but sufficient snugness to stay put?

2. Will they be comfortable if you are lying on a pillow?

3. Do the speakers go inside your ears or over the outsides? Either way, will they be comfortable if you roll onto your side?

4. Is the sound well contained? Can your sleep partner hear it? Some people have reported music sounds traveling through the mattress and bothering their partner.

5. Do you need one set for sleeping and a different style for car or airplane travel?

Unless you are terribly picky about your sound quality, I recommend an inexpensive headset. They are easily replaced if damaged in transit or during a particularly tossy-turny night. I often break or lose mine, so I buy inexpensive sets.

There is one inevitable problem with using headphones. There usually comes a time when you want to remove them, but it's difficult to do that without waking yourself. If you want to avoid the hassle of having to remove your headphones, consider using the pillow speakers described in the next section.

Try a sound pillow or pillow speaker

A big problem with using headphones is the danger of sleeping with a cord. I used to put on the headset and try to stay still to avoid getting tangled, but as we all know, trying to be still can bring on an RLS attack. My problem was solved when I started using a sound pillow.

A sound pillow does not actually have sound of its own. It must be plugged into an audio source (e.g., CD player, TV, cassette player, radio). The pillow will be a relatively normal one, except for the tiny speaker(s) right in the center of all the padding, and the wires leading to the music source. You can still get tangled in the cord if you are not careful, but you will be free to toss and turn without wrapping yourself up in a headset cord.

When you lay on a sound pillow, you shouldn't feel the speakers. With some pillows, you can search for the speakers and press your ear against them. If you can't find the speakers in your pillow, turn up the volume until you hear where they are. Most sound pillows have a definite top and bottom. You will want to figure out which way the speakers are pointing so the sound goes into your ear and not into the mattress. You can also move away from the sounds when you are done listening but are too tired to reach up and shut off the player.

There are some disadvantages to a sound pillow. If you prefer a certain type of pillow, you may not like a sound pillow's firmness or texture. If you take your sound pillow on trips, it takes up a good deal of packing room, and they are relatively expensive at $30–60. Mine is a pretty good basic pillow, but I eventually got tired of stuffing it into my suitcase when I traveled. Before you spend money on a sound pillow, try headphones and make sure you can use music as a reliable and effective RLS trick. You can also achieve the same effect by using an inexpensive pillow speaker. These individual speakers can be found on the Internet or at an electronics store, and cost $4–10. The speaker can be slipped under your pillow (inside the pillow case) with the cord coming out and attaching to your player. Some speakers have volume adjustments and other controls. These features are nice, as long as you can still rest your head on the pillow without feeling the knobs. A pillow speaker can easily be packed in a suitcase and used with any pillow.

Explore other audio options

There are hundreds of options when it comes to picking your audio selections. If you use audio books, consider whether the story is fast-paced and creates good *bully noise*, or so slow that it is a loud invitation to the *RLS bully*. Consider the tone of the narrator's voice. Will a deep mellow voice put you to sleep best, or would a shrill voice create the *bully noise* you need?

If you use a sound machine, be aware that some of them create quiet or sporadic sounds that might relax most people, but might send an RLSer into a fit. You might want to look for a sound machine that produces white noise, which is louder, more complex, and better at keeping your brain from focusing on the useless RLS signals. Sounds of strong winds or constant ocean waves might be more effective than sporadic sounds of birds chirping or frogs croaking. The sound of a room air conditioner or heater can provide excellent noise. You might want to look for sound machines or CDs (used to help colicky babies get to sleep) with the sounds of clothes dryers or vacuum cleaners.

When it comes to music, your options are endless. I prefer songs that are fast-paced. Classical piano music is excellent. I also like to use rock opera and soundtracks from musicals I have enjoyed seeing. As I listen, I can imagine the scenes described in the words of the songs. Figure out what types of music work best for you. Does an instrumental calm you or do you concentrate better when you hear lyrics? Do certain instruments attract your attention more than others? Do not assume you need slow, soft music. Loud and crazy may be the best.

In addition to the type of music and its volume, consider the organization and content of the album. I do better with a combination of sound, speed, and volume. For me, it is best if the first song is loud and fast and the second song is softer and slower. The first one helps draw my attention away from other noises and thoughts. It acts as *bully noise,* overpowering any RLS symptoms. The second song, if it is slower and quieter, seems to set me adrift and allows me to fall into a deep sleep. What amazes me is that the other loud songs on the album do not wake me up again. I seldom remember hearing them.

Do not analyze your musical options while you are trying to get to sleep.

If you are thinking, "I don't like this music, maybe I should try the other album," you will be distracted from your concentration.

Discipline yourself to stay focused rather than allowing your mind to analyze whether it's the best choice of music. In the morning, when you are fresh and not pressured to get to sleep, you can objectively think about different audio selections.

If you are listening to the whole album rather than falling asleep, you may need a completely different type of music. If the music is too familiar or too unfamiliar, you may be listening passively, instead of actively. It does not work to use it as background music for your thoughts. The music must *consume* your thoughts and draw your attention to the music so you can focus and concentrate.

Listen analytically and intently

When listening to music, concentrate on every detail. Try to determine what instruments are producing the sounds. Imagine the movement and expressions of the singers. Soundtracks from musicals, movies, and music videos are nice because they often bring to mind scenes you can easily visualize.

Experiment with the volume until you find a level that helps you stay focused. Sometimes I play music loudly, so the sounds overpower my thoughts and help me stay focused. There are other times when it is best if I lower the volume until it is difficult to hear. When the volume is low, I have to force myself to be very still, press my ear to the speaker, and focus intently on every sound. When the volume is low, I feel as if I am merging with the speaker and getting right into the middle of the music.

When I listen to an album, I seem to fall asleep in stages. I do not worry if I am still aware of the music after the first or second song. I seem to make the most progress during the breaks between songs, trusting that with each break, I will drift a little deeper toward sleep.

Don't resist

It is common to resist what we know will work. Even though I know the best way to get to sleep is to stick to my plan and listen to the music, I sometimes skip that step and try going straight to sleep. It makes me mad that I have to go through all the steps and work so hard at going to sleep. Sometimes I can still get to sleep, even if I skip the music, but sometimes I just waste valuable time and invite RLS symptoms. Shortcuts are not good when you are learning to develop your concentration skills. Follow your plan and learn the discipline of the trick.

The trouble with resisting the plan or using shortcuts, especially when I was first learning these skills, was that by the time I realized I had to start at the beginning and do it all correctly, my RLS was raging. Once the RLS was out of control, it made the whole task of getting to sleep much harder. I am not sure why I tend to resist what I know will work. Maybe it is just my own little protest against the unfairness of having RLS. I almost always end up biting the bullet and going back to a trick I know will work. It boils down to one thing: "If I want to sleep, I have to follow the plan."

Record your techniques

As you develop the skill of using audio for getting to sleep or for staying still during an at-rest activity, remember to write down all the variables that make it work for you. Initially, you will find it is important to follow every detail of your plan. Over time, you may simplify the plan, skip some steps, and change your approach. In fact, you may change it from a prop trick, where you use CD players, headphones, and speaker pillows, to a no-prop trick of just imagining the sounds in your head. As long as you are successfully getting to sleep or sitting still, it will be fine to not follow every detail of your original plan.

As time goes on, various things may aggravate your RLS symptoms and cause you to have to return to the detailed, step-by-step plans you originally developed and recorded. You may want to go back to using headphones, sound pillows, or audio books. By the time you need them again, you may have forgotten all the things you discovered about how to make them work effectively for you. So write them down—now. Make notes about what type of music, what volume, what players, and what sounds work best. You can keep all these notes in your file system, under the section for your Bag of Tricks Approach (BOTA), in either the Gather Your Tricks section or the Plan of Attack section.

Prop Tricks: Non-Prescription

PROP TRICKS ARE therapies or treatments that require the use of a physical object. Examples of prop tricks include prescription medicines, over-the-counter medicines, and various self-help gadgets. This chapter deals with props that do not require a prescription. Prescription medications will be discussed in the following chapter.

There are many advantages to using prop tricks. Many of us prefer treatments we can see and easily apply. When we are sleep deprived and frustrated, it is easier to grab a sucker, plug in a massager, make a cup of tea, or take supplements than to work on learning no-prop tricks like concentration. Props that are inexpensive and easy to obtain can be popular tools to fight Restless Legs Syndrome (RLS). Nevertheless, before getting into a more detailed description of prop tricks, it is worth considering their possible drawbacks. Disadvantages are not mentioned to discourage use, but to remind you to not rely exclusively on prop tricks. Continue to develop your no-prop tricks, which will always be available, safe, no cost, and a great addition to your Bag of Tricks (BOT).

Potential disadvantages of prop tricks

One potential disadvantage of prop tricks is that you might find yourself in the middle of an RLS attack but without the props you need to respond to the symptoms. If you need suckers in order to sit through a movie, you must remember to take suckers to the theater. If you need herbal teas in order to get through a plane trip, you must remember to have them in your carry-on bag. You must plan ahead or you could be left feeling helpless and unable to endure the irresistible urges to wiggle.

A second potential disadvantage is that you might discover a prop has a dead battery or that you consumed the prop during your last RLS attack. If you use consumable props (e.g., suckers, pills, teas), always replace what you use. You may have to keep a supply of batteries or other accessories needed for proper use of certain props.

The third potential disadvantage of prop tricks is that they can cost more than you are willing or able to spend. Though many prop tricks are inexpensive, you can easily spend a small fortune on gadgets and therapies that promise to bring relief. The more the advertisements promise and the more testimonials they give, the more we tend to justify the cost. In most cases, I do not believe a prop trick needs to be expensive to be effective. A later chapter will deal with tips for determining whether a therapy is worth the cost or investment of your time and effort.

Finally, be aware of the potential physical dangers of prop tricks. Herbs, aromatic oils, and mechanical devices can require caution in order to avoid negative effects. Just because the therapy is available without a prescription does not mean it is absolutely safe. The best way to avoid the dangers of prop tricks is to be educated in their safety precautions. Another precaution is to not overuse a particular prop trick. My motto about using any RLS trick is: "Everything in moderation, nothing to excess, and when in doubt, use several tricks and keep the *RLS bully* confused."

Choosing your prop tricks

When conventional medical treatments are combined with other types of treatments, they are referred to as "complementary medicines." Prop tricks can be divided into five categories, commonly used to describe treatments used in complementary medicines: 1) alternative medical systems, 2) biologically-based treatments, 3) manipulative and body-based methods, 4) mind/body interventions, and 5) energy therapies. The next sections of this chapter will mention popular RLS prop tricks in each category. I do not necessarily use, claim the effectiveness of, nor recommend the tricks mentioned in this chapter. The order in which they are listed has nothing to do with how effective I think they might be. Use the information to spark your interest and to give you a taste of what is available. I encourage you to do research, think creatively, and carefully build a personal BOT with your favorite approaches, using prop and no-prop tricks—and always to be aware of potential dangers and costs.

Alternative medical systems

There are many medical systems to consider in addition to the conventional system known in the United States. Other cultures have their own conventional medicines (e.g., traditional Chinese medicines, India's Ayurveda). Oriental cultures have provided us with practices, such as Qi gong, Reiki, and acupuncture. From Western cultures, some RLSers have found temporary relief using chiropractics, homeopathics, and naturopathics.

Alternative medical treatments might alleviate a physical or mental condition that aggravates your RLS. As an indirect result, you might experience relief from your RLS symptoms. However, even though your headache, backache, or other RLS-aggravating condition was relieved, there may be other aggravators that will trigger the next RLS attack. As long as you realize that alternative treatments are only relieving RLS aggravators and not providing permanent RLS relief, you probably won't be disappointed.

Biologically-based treatments

Biologically-based substances include those found in nature, as well as those that are man-made. When you address your deficiencies in Step 4 of the Reduction Plan, you may decide to use some biologically-based prop tricks, such as vitamins, minerals, herb complexes, or changes in your diet. The following are some potentially useful biologically-based props:

Non-prescription medicines: Many over-the-counter medicines previously required prescriptions and should be treated with the same caution and intelligence as prescription medicines. Many people report relief from something as common as acetaminophen (e.g., Tylenol). Problems can arise, however, if a person takes a product that combines acetaminophen with an antihistamine (e.g., Tylenol PM). The antihistamine can actually aggravate RLS symptoms rather than producing the desired effect of inducing sleep. Do your research and become educated about the safety and precautions of any over-the-counter medicines you use.

DHA/Neuromins: DHA is an omega-3 essential fatty acid. It is normally sold as fish oil, but it is also available as a vegetarian supplement containing alagal oil, high oleic sunflower oil, vitamin C, vitamin E, and beta-carotene in a gelatin capsule. This vegetarian source of DHA goes by the patented name of DHA/Neuromins. My experience with DHA has been with Neuromins, but the same benefits might be possible with the fish oil form of DHA.

During my early search for helpful supplements, someone emailed me his story of obtaining RLS relief from DHA/Neuromins. While taking DHA/Neuromins for a heart condition, he noticed his RLS symptoms had practically disappeared. When his pregnant daughter followed her doctor's recommendation to take DHA/Neuromins, she reported a similar decrease in her RLS symptoms. I was intrigued by these stories. In my research, the only danger I saw was if someone were to use the fish oil form of DHA, which is often sold in combination with EPA, another omega-3 fatty acid. Because EPA can act as a blood thinner, it would be contra-indicated if a person were already taking prescription blood thinners or certain heart medications. (There is a possibility the vitamin E in DHA/Neuromins might also create a problem with someone trying to avoid blood thinners.)

When I began taking DHA/Neuromins, I experienced a steady decrease in the severity of my RLS symptoms. Taking more DHA/Neuromins did not make it better, but taking less definitely increased the frequency and severity of my RLS symptoms. With some experimentation, I settled on a dose that has continued to work for me. By "work for me," I mean it decreases the severity of my RLS so I can manage the rest with my usual BOT, but it does not prevent RLS symptoms. Some RLSers have positive results with DHA/Neuromins, while others find it makes no difference. As always, each of us must find what our unique system needs. Please remember, I try to not recommend one brand of a product, but in this case, DHA/Neuromins is the only form of DHA I have tried. I shared this story to give you an idea of some of the thoughts that led me to try some of my supplements, not because I think you should use the product.

Aromas: The use of aromas for RLS therapy can be as simple as breathing a pleasant smell. On the other hand, it can be as complex as carefully administering therapeutic doses of essential oils. I have been told there are ways to cause problems with misused aroma therapy. Therefore, I would only recommend a very simplistic use of aromas, unless you are knowledgeable in this area.

When I use aroma therapy, my goal is to find an aroma that makes me feel good and encourages me to take deep, relaxing breaths. When I use anything with a sweet jasmine smell (e.g., candle, oils, perfumes) I have pleasurable memories of being in Hawaii. I instantly smile, breathe deeply, and relax. The same smell might produce completely opposite results for someone else. As always, you must safely experiment and find what works for you.

Herbal teas: Celestial Seasoning's Tension Tamer tea has calmed my legs on many occasions. Many other RLSers have also found it helpful, but as with all RLS tricks, there are people who say it does not help them at all. There are even those who say they can't stand the taste of it. There is a *wellness variety* by the same name (sold in drugstores), but the ingredients are slightly different. I get better results from the original one, in the blue box, sold in grocery stores. Again, I am not suggesting the brand I use is the one you should choose. I am merely using this brand as an example, because it's a product I have tried and used successfully. If you do not want to use Tension Tamer tea, you might consider looking for something with similar ingredients or claiming to be relaxing or sleep inducing.

When using an herbal tea medicinally, you need to prepare it properly for the results you intend. Just a few dunks of a tea bag in the hot water will probably not produce medicinal results. I use two bags of tea in two cups of water and let it steep for five to ten minutes. Read the directions that come with your herbal tea. Some prefer that you do not allow the water to boil. I leave the bags in the water until I slowly sip the last strong medicinal drop of tea. I get the best results if I drink it slowly while I am engrossed in a computer game. I haven't had much success with it overpowering an RLS attack while I am watching television, but it does work well for me when traveling on airplanes (see "Traveler's RLS").

The following are additional tips to consider when using herbal teas or herbal supplements.

1. **Treat herbal teas and supplements as medicine.** If you are using herbs to produce specific results, you are us-

ing them as medicine. Learn to use safe doses and appropriate varieties.

2. **Target specific results.** Just as you would want to know the purpose and effects of prescription drugs, you should also know what to expect from herbs. Tension Tamer tea will calm my legs, but will not make me sleepy. If I want to encourage sleepiness, I might add a bag of chamomile tea.

3. **Consider using blends.** Rather than using a specific herb by itself, I prefer to use commercial blends. I feel more confident about getting the amount I need, along with other herbs that might enhance the results. For example, rather than drinking a straight valerian or chamomile tea, you might find one called Sleep Tonight (a fictitious name) that might be a nice blend of sleep-inducing herbs.

4. **Identify possible negative results:** Some herbs can produce unwanted results. They might duplicate the purpose of a prescription medication you are taking. More importantly, they might have negative interactions with another medicine. Even with a tea blend, you might find one of the herbs can cause unfavorable reactions. As always, do your research and proceed with caution. It's always a good idea to discuss what you are using with your doctor.

5. **Consider the source:** Be concerned about the manufacturer and source of the herbs. I tend to prefer relatively inexpensive, but well-known brands of teas and herbs.

Herbal supplements: When trying herbal supplements, apply the tips for using herbal teas (see above). It is not always convenient to use herbal teas. Some people prefer to quickly swallow supplements in pill form. Others insist a tincture (alcohol solution) form is the only way to go. As always, do your research and treat your herbal supplements as medicines. Be careful of potential side effects and interactions with other medications. Valerian, kava kava, and chamomile are just a few of the popular herbal supplements used for relaxation and sleep.

Folic Acid, calcium, vitamin E, and iron: These supplements are all commonly suggested for reducing severity and frequency of RLS symptoms. There are many risks in suggesting supplementation. Not all of us have the same deficiencies. Many of these supplements come in different forms and different combinations, so a decision to try a vitamin or mineral is only the beginning.

You must also ask, "How much? How often? When should it be taken? Are there dangers?"

Supplements vary greatly. I have tried two different calcium supplements from the same company, with almost identical amounts of calcium, but the results were very different. Experiment carefully, preferably under the supervision of your doctor, and educate yourself before you start using supplemental pills.

Do not give up on a supplement after trying it once. You may be able to adjust dosages, combinations, manufacturers, and timing. A supplement's absorption ability and effectiveness can be affected by many things, including the presence or absence of other nutrients. You could think you didn't need a supplement you tried, when in fact, it was never absorbed into your system because you were low on nutrients that were essential for its absorption.

A supplement may appear to be ineffective if too many other aggravators are making RLS symptoms go crazy. When the aggravators are removed and the beast is back to bully size, the supplements may become effective. Once you decide that you have found a supplement you need, experiment with whether more is better or whether you can take less and get the same good results. Make changes slowly and keep good notes.

"Miracle" drinks and supplements: I refer to these as "miracle" drinks and supplements because they are usually advertised as having miraculous results for almost any ailment you can imagine. Often, these products are sold through a multi-level marketing system. We used to call them pyramid schemes until pyramid programs were outlawed and the businesses made changes to stay legal. High-pressure sales techniques often include testimonials from others who claim they suffered from your ailment but found relief with a certain miracle product. In light of all the claims of relief, it's easy to feel guilty for not trying the product. Here's my advice. Look at the ingredients of the products. There is a good chance they are filled with vitamins and nutrients that are not unique to that product. You might be able to try some of those ingredients on your own and zero in on something your body needs.

I found one product used a *sea plant.* Knowing the DHA/Neuromins I use is made from marine plants, it makes sense the product might help my RLS. But why use it, when I'm already using DHA/Neuromins?

Just remember, miracle drinks and supplements are not miraculous cures. They might address some of your deficiencies and they might give you more energy. This alone might reduce the severity of your RLS. They can definitely be a useful prop in your BOT, if used with realistic expectations.

Manipulative and body-based methods

Some prop tricks are designed to stimulate muscles, increase circulation, distract you with movement, calm you, or stimulate your nerves. Consider some of the following options and whether they might provide relief for you.

Massage: There are many kinds of massage. Just because someone tried to rub your legs and it didn't work, don't give up on massage. There are times when the base of my hand, pushed up and down my thigh, relieves the RLS symptoms and the tightened muscles resulting from an RLS attack. At other times, a fast light-pressured rubbing works best, distracting my mind as the quick rubbing builds friction and provides lingering warmth. If someone else is providing your massage, be sure to communicate by telling the person what you need, where you need it, and how to make it more effective. It might be helpful to provide feedback by using a numbering system. For instance:

10 . . . Stop now! It hurts!

8 . . . Lighten up! It may be OK, if you ease into it.

6 . . . You found a tender area. Continue cautiously.

4–5 . . . It feels just right. Keep it up for about three hours. Don't wake me when you're done.

1–3 . . . What's the point? I can barely feel it.

Vibrators and massagers: Be aware of various types of mechanical massagers. Some of them go back and forth rapidly; others provide heat. Percussive massagers pound up and down on the muscles. As always, analyze your symptoms and choose the treatment that makes the most sense. Above all, guard your finances. Many expensive gadgets have equally effective inexpensive look-alikes. I paid over $200 for a percussive massager, only to find I could have gotten one exactly like it for $40. I even bought the $40 model and blindfolded myself while my husband used both models on my legs. I could not tell the difference.

There are many varieties of heated and non-heated vibrating seat cushions. These can be very helpful during long car trips. They are also nice to use in a recliner, when you are watching TV, reading, or trying to nap.

Some RLSers find it useful to put a vibrating pillow under their desk and keep their feet on it while they work at the computer. At first, the sensations may trigger more RLS, but once the person gets used to the feeling, it can be very relaxing.

Machines that move you: There are numerous products that stimulate circulation by moving your body for you. Some machines swing your legs back and forth while you passively lie on your back. Others stimulate circulation in your limbs by creating pulsating pressure. If you do an Internet search for "foot stimulation massage machines," you will be amazed at the available products. Before you buy anything, read the chapter, "Is It Worth a Try?" If you are not sure about a gadget, consider looking for a used one at a garage sale or on the Internet. If you decide to buy a new product, make sure there is a good refund policy.

For years, hospitals have used various devices to stimulate circulation in the legs of surgery patients. One of the more popular machines has pads that are wrapped around the legs and hoses that periodically pump the pads full of air. The squeezing motion stimulates blood circulation and prevents clots, swelling, and other problems caused by prolonged bed rest. Similar compression units are now available for personal purchase.

Ask yourself, "Will I take the time to put them on? Will I be able to stay still and allow them to work?"

There are several types of units which use electricity to stimulate muscles. The prices on these tend to be pretty high, but if you ask around, you might find someone who has one they will loan you. With correct application and the right type of unit, you might find you like this trick.

Gadgets you move: You can buy a two-chambered pillow, usually sold to stimulate blood circulation for people on long airplane trips. You place the pillow under your feet and alternately press on the left and right sides, forcing the air through a small channel connecting one chamber to the other. If you want to get a feel for how these pillows work, try putting both feet on the floor and alternately pressing them down. You should feel it in your thighs, as if you were walking. If this motion works for you, maybe you do not need to buy the pillow. Maybe it will become a perfect no-prop trick.

Similar to the two-chambered pillows, are the stepper/walker units. These are usually two foot pedals that you press alternately to simulate walking movements while you remain seated. Some are extremely compact and can be slipped into a purse or pocket.

Another gadget you move is a pedal/cycle exerciser. If you have RLS in your arms, you might use the exerciser on a table top, dispelling RLS symptoms by moving the pedals with your hands. It can also be placed on the floor, pedaled by foot, and used for RLS symptoms in legs. There have even been cases of people using them in vehicles (e.g., sitting in the back of a van or RV and pedaling cross country while someone else did the driving).

Water: Hot tubs, bathtubs, and hot showers are well known as useful therapies for RLSers.

Stretching devices: Many devices which exercise limbs and muscles will indirectly relieve RLS symptoms. One of the cheapest and simplest tricks is to use a therapy band. These large rubber or latex bands can be positioned around the ball of the foot and pulled on while you flex your foot and stretch your calves. They are very handy in cars, air-planes, theaters, or if you have to sit through long lectures or meetings. The advantage of what I call the *rubber band trick* is that you can stay seated and keep concentrating on what's going on. Also, the bands are small enough to always have with you, just in case. They can be purchased from some medical supply stores. You might also obtain one from an aerobics instructor or physical therapist.

Sex: A thousand disclaimers! Be responsible! If you have a safe way to enjoy sex, don't hesitate to consider it as one of the best manipulative and body-based tricks. Of course, it could also fit in the categories of mind-body interventions. There's nothing quite like it when it comes to movement (for some people), focusing your mind (okay, not for everyone) and energy (does it give it or drain it?). Needless-to-say, the use of sex as an RLS treatment will be different for everyone. I also mentioned this trick in the chapter on no-prop tricks. You can decide where it belongs.

Mind-body interventions

If you learn to do mind-body intervention on your own, it may fall under the category of no-prop tricks (e.g., concentration, *bully noise*). Many prop tricks focus on getting our thoughts to intervene and actually change certain bodily functions and symptoms. In some cases, the goal is to distract our minds from the RLS urges. In other situations, the emphasis is on reducing RLS symptoms by reducing anxiety.

We cringe when we hear someone say, "Just relax. It's all in your mind."

Though we know RLS survival is far more complicated than just relaxing and having all the symptoms go away, there is some wisdom in looking at how we can adjust our thoughts and positively influence our RLS survival.

Support groups: People can be a wonderful prop if they share the same frustrations and are working toward achieving the same results. RLS support groups can be found in almost every state of the United States, as well as in several foreign countries. Contact information for support groups can be found on the Restless Legs Syndrome Foundation website (http://www.rls.org). The RLS Foundation will be happy to help people start their own local support group. There are also virtual support groups, where people post letters on the Internet and share ideas. My favorite Internet group has been at http://groups.yahoo.com. If you wish to try it, search for a group called "rlssupport." Many new group members have reported instant improvement in their RLS symptoms after discovering they were not the only ones experiencing them. The group's support and the newly acquired RLS information create a mental change that often brings quick improvement.

Spiritual therapy: Spiritual therapies can enhance an RLSer's ability to deal successfully with RLS. Whereas prayer and meditation can easily be considered no-prop tricks, other spiritual therapies may require props (e.g., reading the bible, prayer groups, spiritual counseling). At the very least, spiritual therapies can be helpful in avoiding the depression and disillusionment that can come from sleep deprivation and constant bombardment of RLS symptoms.

Psychological or psychiatric therapy: In many cases, it helps to understand your own thinking and analyze what is influencing your mind and body. I am sure I have conscious and subconscious thoughts that influence or trigger some of my RLS symptoms. Mental therapy may not be the whole answer, but why not address every area? If you decide to use psychiatric counseling, be careful about recommendations to take anti-depressants. Do some research and learn about the potential negative effects some anti-depressants have on RLS.

Music: The previous chapter was devoted to the use of music as a way to prevent, diminish or overpower RLS symptoms.

Crafts and hobbies: Many RLSers find it helpful to do a craft or hobby while trying to remain still. Knitting, needlework, playing cards, painting, computer work, and playing a musical instrument are all activities that involve focusing or distracting your mind in an attempt to deal with RLS symptoms.

Hypnosis: Whether you practice hypnosis with a therapist (prop trick), or learn to do self-hypnosis (no-prop trick), the benefits can be worth your time. Ideally, this will become a no-prop trick you can use wherever you are, but it may initially require music, machines, or the help of another person.

Pillow speakers: Pillow speakers and sound pillows were discussed in the previous chapter on using music. These were two of my favorite and most effective props during the first years I consciously fought back against RLS.

Suckers, peanuts, popcorn, and raisins: People kid me about my suckers, because I swear they distract me and allow me to finish many at-rest activities, despite RLS symptoms. I laugh about them, too. I've settled on one brand I like best and I try to always have them in my BOT. The brand I like is made by Tootsie and sold mostly around Halloween. They are Caramel Apple Pops. Mmm! Maybe they are just a placebo or maybe they just keep me busy. Perhaps the sweet and sour flavors confuse my brain and keep it too busy to send RLS signals. I don't know why the suckers work so well, but a reason is not important, as long as they keep working. (Reminder: I am not promoting this brand. Choose your own favorite sucker. Disclaimer: I am not responsible for your dental bill. Warning: Do not use this prop trick for going to sleep at night.)

Other foods can help by distracting our minds and keeping us moving as we slowly pop them into our mouths. Popcorn, peanuts, and raisins are popular tricks many RLSers insist on having whenever they attempt to sit still for a play, movie, or concert. Popcorn is an important part of my ability to sit still and enjoy a movie in a public theater.

I had to laugh when I saw a "Family Circus" cartoon in our newspaper, where Dolly was saying, "I love it when we go out for a big tub of popcorn and see a movie."

Because the pre-show advertisements and trailers take up so much time, I have to be careful to save the popcorn for the start of the movie.

Energy therapies

There are two main types of energy therapies to consider. One type works with alleged energy fields that exist in and around our bodies. Certain types of massage and therapeutic touch therapies address these fields. Acupuncture and acupressure also manipulate energy fields. Another type involves applying electromagnetic fields to the body. There are machines that do this, but the treatments can be quite costly. I have used magnets for strains to muscles and tendons, and I am pretty sure they were effective. If those ailments aggravated my RLS, it would make sense to use magnets as an indirect therapy for RLS. However, I am not convinced they work directly against whatever causes RLS symptoms.

Some people will argue there is a difference in which magnets you use, which way they point, and how you use them. I have been approached by company representatives who swear that regular use of their expensive electromagnetic machines or magnetic mattress pads would cure me of RLS. Magnetic therapy may be just the thing for you, but just like with every trick, you have to use it intelligently. Before you rush out and buy expensive magnetic pads and devices, ask your friends and family if they have similar products you can borrow and try. As always, do research, make careful choices, and have realistic expectations.

I have seen comments in legitimate RLS brochures and bulletins saying there are studies being done to test the effectiveness of certain magnetic or energy field treatments. With more research, you may find some promising new treatments have become available since I wrote this book.

The *bar of soap trick*
Effective prop or placebo?

One of the most frequently cited tricks for dealing with RLS symptoms is the *bar of soap trick*. It is so popular, I decided to give it a section of its own. The claim is that RLS symptoms will be prevented if you place a bar of soap at the foot of your bed, under the fitted sheet. Some people claim certain brands of soap work better than others. I can't tell you how many times someone has told me they know the cure for RLS, and then proceeded to explain the *bar of soap trick*. I have even received bars of soap wrapped as gifts from well meaning people who were excited about giving me an easy cure for a problem that has plagued me for years.

In many cases where people have sworn the *bar of soap trick* worked for them, they were reporting cases of muscle cramps or PLMS (Periodic Limb Movements of Sleep) rather than RLS symptoms. After hearing many reports of RLSers trying this trick and saying it was ineffective, I am pretty convinced any positive results are a placebo effect.

RLS tricks are thought to provide a placebo effect when they provide temporary relief without a known reason. Many people treat the placebo effect as a bad thing. A placebo effect might be the result of a person's faith in the treatment. It could derive from the excitement of trying something new. Benefits can come from the act of preparing the trick (i.e., going to the kitchen and making tea). The way I see it, any safely provided relief is worth considering, especially if it is inexpensive.

As of the printing of this book, there is an excellent website (http://www.rlshelp.org) that lists and discusses many props people claim are helpful in relieving their RLS. If the site is still available, you will find seemingly endless ideas of props to consider, along with a doctor's review of the various ideas.

Keep searching

The props I've discussed in this chapter are only a sample of what you might consider having in your BOT. Keep researching and finding new ideas. Remember to consider new and effective ways to use props you already have. You may have been unsuccessful in your attempts to use a certain prop because your RLS was still too far out of control. After you apply the Reduction Plan and minimize the severity of your RLS, that same prop might become effective. You may have had unsuccessful results from one type of massage, only to find another type works perfectly. Keep learning, searching, and re-evaluating, so you always have a useful supply of prop tricks for your BOT.

Prop Tricks: Prescription

Disclaimer: I am not qualified to give specific advice on prescription medications. Please discuss the use of pharmaceuticals with your doctor. This chapter will suggest thoughts and attitudes about incorporating prescription drugs in your Bag of Tricks (BOT). It will also give a brief description of the types of drugs commonly used to combat RLS symptoms.

Start your research

EVEN IF YOU do not plan to use prescription medications, it is a good idea to learn about them. If a sudden need for medications arises, it will help if you are already well informed and ready to make educated choices about your treatment. It is best to learn about prescription medications before you are too sleep deprived to make sense of the information.

In your research, you will find information about drugs and their side effects. You will also find terminology which you will want to learn. Many drugs cause rebound (a shorter time when each dose is effective) or augmentation (when the Restless Legs Syndrome [RLS] symptoms begin attacking earlier in the day or in other parts of the body). These terms are easy to confuse, but important to understand. Later in this chapter, I will mention four categories of drugs used for RLS treatments. Make it part of your self-education to become familiar with the differences in the names of the categories: dopaminergics, benzodiazepines, opioids, and anticonvulsants.

Some RLSers opt to use prescription drugs for isolated situations where they need extra assistance (e.g., during a long plane trip, when facing surgery, while dealing with the aftermath of a traumatic event). By starting their research early and keeping abreast of new information, they can always be ready for those special RLS-provoking situations.

Information on pharmaceutical treatments is constantly changing. Feedback from RLSers is altering what we thought we knew about current pharmaceutical RLS treatments. At the same time, new drugs are being introduced and we are learning how they can be effective in relieving RLS symptoms. It is much easier to grasp new information when you already have a good foundation of research and education about the pharmaceuticals already being used for RLS.

Keep good notes

Keep records of what you find in your research about RLS pharmaceutical treatments. You can store pharmaceutical information in the Bag of Tricks Approach (BOTA) Step 1: Gather Your Tricks section of your notebook. You can include copies of brochures, articles, printouts of website material, and notes about your own experiences with various pharmaceuticals.

If you are already using pharmaceuticals, take the drugstore's printed material on each drug and store it in your notebook with your research notes. Add personal notes about the benefits and drawbacks of the drug. As time goes on, you might change your dosages from what the drugstore printout states. Be sure to record how your usage of the drug changes. If you don't have pre-printed information on drugs, you can make your own fact sheet template with some of the following points:

1. Name of drug or generic name of drug.

2. Category of drug (dopaminergic agent, opioid, benzodiazepine, anticonvulsant).

3. Expected results (induce sleep, stop RLS symptoms, reduce anxiety, etc.).

4. Advantages (goes to work quickly, can be taken *as needed*, does not cause drowsiness, etc.).

5. Disadvantages (causes insomnia, takes a while to start working, can cause augmentation or rebound).

6. Cost (Is it covered by your insurance?)

7. Recommended dosage for RLS (Is there a recommended maximum dose for RLS?)

Reasons to postpone pharmaceutical use

If you decide to use pharmaceuticals, you should do so with commitment and resolve that it is the best choice at the time. As you consider whether it is a good time to start using pharmaceuticals, be aware of realistic reasons to postpone their use. There is no rule or goal that says you should never use drugs as RLS treatments, but there are some personal preferences and considerations that might suggest you postpone their use or keep your pharmaceutical tricks to a minimum. I will share some of my own preferences as examples.

Obviously, prescription medications can be expensive and time-consuming. By the time you go to the doctor, fill the prescription, and manage your insurance papers, you have invested a good deal of time. If I can successfully use self-help tricks and not have to invest the extra time and money in using pharmaceuticals, I will.

Another consideration for me is my family history. Several members of my family have had illnesses or ailments that caused them to take a large number of prescription medications. With that kind of family history, I have always figured it is just a matter of time before I will need them, too. The fewer drugs I take now, the less concern I will have with drug interactions if I need to add others to my list of treatments.

Wear and tear on my organs has always been a concern for me. I know many prescription drugs create physical problems of their own. When I was diagnosed with ovarian cancer in 2005, it was very nice to hear all my organs were in great shape and I would easily tolerate the surgery and chemotherapy treatments that followed. I decided I might not be able to prevent some illnesses, but I could do my best to keep my body in good shape to fight back against anything I might experience.

These are just considerations. They do not rule out the possibility I might use prescription medications to treat my RLS along the way.

Rebellious thoughts about pharmaceuticals

Despite the personal concerns I just gave, I am actually in favor of using prescription drugs for RLS. That statement will raise the eyebrows of some readers. Many people think of me as being in favor of only alternative approaches, but this is far from true. As you read more about "rebel thinking" on using drugs for RLS, you will understand how I can say I am in favor of pharmaceutical treatments, even though I do not currently use them myself.

Though I am in favor of using prescription drugs, I am still opposed to some common thoughts about using drugs for RLS treatment.

I worry when I hear someone say, "I am going to the doctor today, and he'd better fix me," because that person is assuming there is already a *fix* available.

I am also concerned when someone says, "I deserve to be able to take a pill and not have to deal with RLS."

We all deserve and hope for this, but is it realistic to expect it?

In order to effectively incorporate prescription medications into your BOTA, it will help to contrast some common ways of thinking about drugs with some new ways of thinking about pharmaceutical treatments for RLS. Some common thoughts about prescription drug use set the patient up for disappointment and hamper the success of drug treatments. The following sections will give you an idea of how a slight change to "rebel thoughts" can help pharmaceutical use be a valuable part of your BOT.

Drugs are *wimping out* or drugs are *assisted living*

Common thinking: "I give up. Maybe I'm *wimping out*, but I just can't do it on my own."

Rebel thinking: "I need more assistance and more options in my BOTA. Prescription medication might be just the extra help I need right now."

The decision to use the assistance of prescription medications for RLS can emotionally devastate some people, making them feel as if they are *wimping out* and giving up. For other people, a decision to try pharmaceuticals can encourage them and boost their morale. It is similar to the decision many elderly people make about whether to live in an assisted living residence or to continue living on their own. Some people become overwhelmed at the difficulties of living on their own. When they move to an assisted living community, they can thrive with fewer worries, a more active social life, and the benefit of available medical attention. Other people might thrive at home, but would feel helpless and would give up if they moved to an assisted living facility.

Just as some people must decide between living on their own or using an assisted living facility, many RLSers must decide whether they should stick to self-help treatments or incorporate the assistance of prescription medications. The decision to use assisted living or the assistance of prescription medications for RLS does not relieve you of control and responsibility to stay in charge of your program. The pill is assistance, not a cure, the same as an assisted living facility provides assistance, not full care.

You can't give up and turn your RLS treatment program over to a doctor, expecting him to fix all your problems and meet all your needs. If you decide to use the assistance of prescription drugs, you must still be very involved in your own care. You will need to manage the drugs, note the side effects, communicate with your doctor, and deal with the costs and other complications of using medications. I hope, you will also be working on the other parts of the RLS Rebel Program—reducing the *beast of RLS* and perfecting your BOTA. A decision to use prescription medications is a decision to become more involved in your survival program, not a decision to wimp out.

Drugs are a *last resort* or drugs can be early intervention

Common thinking: "I think of drugs as a last resort. I will not use them until all other treatments have failed or my RLS is too severe for any alternative tricks."

Rebel thinking: "I might use pharmaceuticals well before my RLS becomes severe."

Early in my experience of sharing ideas about RLS, a fellow RLSer criticized me for being against prescription medications. While trying to assure him I was not saying anything against using prescription medication, I asked where he got that idea.

After long discussions, it boiled down to my always saying, "I hope I will not have to resort to using medications."

The word *resort* gave away thoughts I didn't realize I had. I was definitely thinking of drugs as the treatment I'd use — after I had tried everything else and had basically given up on the idea of being able to deal with RLS on my own.

Similar thinking is still prevalent among medical professionals and many RLSers. They speak of a linear approach, where we try self-help treatments until our RLS is severe, and then we put aside all our alternative treatments and *resort* to pharmaceuticals.

There are many disadvantages to the linear "last resort" approach. Why wait until everything is severe and out of control before considering prescription medications? If you give up on all alternative tricks, rely on just pharmaceuticals, and eventually run out of pharmaceuticals that work, what will be your next option?

I have known several RLSers who swore their RLS was too severe for my rebel tricks. They tried one medication after another until they ran out of options that worked for them. Finally, they asked me to help them incorporate self-help tricks into their program so their medications had a chance to work.

There are many advantages to early intervention with pharmaceutical treatments.

1. In some cases, early intervention with drugs can prevent RLS from becoming more severe. If a person is already sleep deprived and frantic, medications may help him catch up on sleep, successfully apply the steps of the RLS Rebel Program, and gain control.

2. Strategic use of pharmaceuticals might be the answer to making alternative treatments more effective. A person who has used a drug to get a good night of sleep may have a better chance of getting through a workday and handling daytime RLS with alternative tricks. On the contrary, some people need help with pharmaceuticals

during the day, but are able to get to sleep at night on their own.

3. Using drugs while the RLSer is still using alternative measures can help make the drugs effective. A drug that is working against totally out-of-control RLS will have a hard time being effective. When alternative measures and the steps of the Reduction Plan are keeping some of the RLS symptoms minimized, prescription medications have a much better chance of being effective.

4. When pharmaceuticals are introduced early, it gives the RLSer time to recognize side effects, try different medicines, and determine appropriate dosages. When medicines are used against moderate RLS symptoms, the RLSer can probably use lower dosages and avoid the risks of higher dosages of the drugs.

5. By making pharmaceutical use available early in an RLSer's program, the RLSer will be ready for isolated situations that may be more bearable with the assistance of medications (e.g., during long plane trips, when facing surgeries, while dealing with the aftermath of traumatic events).

Drugs make you dependent or drugs keep you independent

Common thinking: "I've tried everything else. I am helpless and dependent on drugs."

Rebel thinking: "I can still get the job done if I incorporate prescription drugs into my BOT."

When I used to refer to drugs as a last resort, I gave many RLSers the impression I thought they had lost all control and had given up their independence by deciding to use prescription drugs. Thanks to their patience with me and their willingness to explain their unique situations, I developed a whole new attitude about using prescription medications. Today, I believe that independence isn't a matter of doing it all by yourself, but a matter of staying in control and getting the job done. If a person gets the job done by using prescription medicine, it does not mean independence has been forfeited. In fact, successful use of prescription drugs is probably more likely when RLSers retain control and feel encouraged by the selection of effective tricks in their BOT.

Drugs cure RLS or drugs relieve RLS symptoms

Common thinking: "Prescription medications will cure my RLS and rid me of all symptoms."

Rebel thinking: "Prescription medicines might provide symptom relief, but I will still have RLS."

Some RLSers find medications that initially seem to rid them of all RLS symptoms. In most cases, however, when asked if the medicine provides 100 percent RLS relief, they will say no. They will describe times when they have *breakthrough* RLS symptoms. For those who claim they have no symptoms, it is often just a matter of time before they change their response and report the return of some RLS symptoms. It is important to realize prescription drugs can dramatically improve an RLSer's quality of life by reducing the severity and frequency of symptoms, but they do not guarantee a symptom-free experience.

If you take an antibiotic for an infection, you can expect to be cured and symptom-free because the antibiotic will kill the bacteria causing the symptoms. This is not the case with RLS medications. Prescription medications might temporarily prevent the irresistible urges to wiggle or help you get to sleep, but you will still have RLS. You can avoid being disappointed in your prescription medication by making sure you are realistic about the results you expect.

The doctor dictates drug use or the patient communicates needs

Common thinking: "My doctor is an RLS specialist. I will let him decide what I need."

Rebel thinking: "I will determine my treatment priorities and communicate these to my doctor. Together, we will develop a pharmaceutical treatment plan that works with my RLS survival program."

A doctor might be called an *RLS specialist* because of his knowledge of RLS, experience in the field, and notoriety among other doctors and organizations focusing on RLS research and treatments, but being an RLS specialist does not mean he will immediately know what treatment is best for you. Working with an RLS specialist will save you the trouble of having to educate your doctor about RLS. It might even mean the doctor has a drug he prefers to try with RLS patients, but you will still have to work as a team to determine the best course of action for your particular situation.

To insure wise use of prescription medicine, there must be clear communications between doctor and patient. This puts a great deal of responsibility on both individuals to explain things well, prioritize needs, and listen carefully to each other.

If you complain about all your symptoms at once, saying, "I'm exhausted, I'm in pain, I can't sit still, I'm depressed, and I haven't slept in weeks," your doctor will have to assess which symptom to treat first. If the doctor decides sleep is the critical issue, a sleeping pill might be prescribed. If you think the critical issue is being able to sit still at your desk, you might be hoping for a medicine that will help you be still. Won't you be surprised if you take the prescription and then you not only can't sit still, but you also can't stay awake? Decide what issues or symptoms are most important to you, and communicate these with your doctor. Together, you can choose the best medicine for you.

RLSers have different needs and priorities. I have heard many RLSers say they can handle their daytime RLS symptoms, but they want to use prescription medicines to help them sleep. I have heard others say they can deal with sleep issues, but they need help getting through daytimes activities (e.g., long carpool rides, classes, meetings). Again, these are issues and concerns that you and the doctor must agree upon before your treatment is decided. Ask questions and be familiar with the intended results of your medication. Know what results to expect and give pertinent feedback to your doctor. Consider some of the following questions.

1. How is the medicine to be used (e.g., dosages and frequency)?
2. Can you safely adjust the dosage on your own?
3. Can you stop taking the medicine *cold turkey?*
4. What should you do if the medicine stops working?
5. What is the medicine supposed to do (e.g., calm you, make you sleepy, relieve depression)?
6. What side effects can you expect?
7. When should you report side effects to your doctor?
8. What does the medicine cost? Are there cheaper options?
9. Can the medicine cause rebound or augmentation?
10. Is the medicine contra-indicated with any of your current physical problems or medications?

There are many drugs to choose from, so do not relinquish your right to be involved in the decision. Work as a team with your doctor and find the best pharmaceutical addition to your BOT.

Use a drug approved for RLS or use the best medications for current needs

Common thinking: "I want the medicine they say is for RLS."

Rebel thinking: "I want the medication which will address my specific needs."

In 2005, Requip became the first drug approved by the FDA for use with RLS. With the approval of Requip, television and news media advertising brought RLS to the attention of thousands who had never heard of the syndrome. It would be easy for people to get the impression there is one special drug that works for all RLS symptoms.

Your doctor may prefer starting with a specific medication that has brought good results with the majority of his RLS patients. It is well known, however, what works for one RLSer will not necessarily work for another. Our chemical make-up and our physical health are different. All of these variables combine to make it so there is no magic answer that fits everyone or every situation.

Rely on drugs or rely on a diverse BOT with pharmaceuticals and alternatives

Common thought: "I don't have time for lots of tricks. I want to take one pill that works."

Rebel thought: "My prescription treatment will be one of many tricks in my full BOT."

An RLSer once wrote to me, "At my age, and as long as I have struggled with RLS, I should not have to use a whole Bag of Tricks. I deserve to be able to take one pill and have the symptoms disappear."

I thought she must be eighty-five years old and she'd probably had RLS since childhood, but I will never forget my shock when I found out she was five years younger than me and had dealt with RLS symptoms for only a few years. I was curious about her insinuation that there actually was one pill that could fix all her RLS problems. Many RLSers have made similar comments, insisting they have no interest in doing a whole BOT when they could take one pill to do the job. The error in their thinking is the idea there is only one job that needs to be done. At one moment, the job might be to get sleep. At another, it might be to sit still and stay alert. My experience with prescription drug use for RLSers is that there is often a need for a combination of drugs that must be periodically adjusted.

There was a time when doctors pushed conventional medicine treatments and scoffed at alternative medicines. Today, complementary medicines are the trend, promoting the benefits of a combined approach. A diverse BOT can provide a complementary medicine approach and give you the most options. Before giving up all your self-help tricks and settling on just using pharmaceuticals, consider some of the following scenarios that might make you wish you had not relied strictly on pharmaceuticals.

1. **We all forget.** What if you went on a vacation and forgot to take your prescription medications with you? What if you went to pack them and suddenly realized you forgot to have your prescription refilled in time for your departure?

2. **Unexpected problems arise.** What if weather problems or an airline strike caused you to be delayed or stranded? What if you couldn't get refills in time?

3. **Refills aren't always possible.** What if you ran out of medications, tried to get a refill, but were told you had to see your doctor first? What if your doctor were out

of town or couldn't fit you into his schedule for several weeks? With some medications, the doctor might prescribe enough to tide you over, but what if you were going to be on a trip for a few months and needed more than he would prescribe without another office visit? What if your prescription were for narcotics (which are often used with RLS) and the doctor, pharmacist, or insurance company suspected misuse and refused to authorize a refill? This has happened to many people. The RLSer becomes caught in the middle while timing, paperwork, and legalities get straightened out. If your prescription medication were the only trick in your bag, you would be out of luck.

4. **Symptoms can suddenly be worse.** What if your RLS suddenly seemed worse, but you didn't want to raise the dosage of your medicines? A sudden worsening of symptoms is often called *breakthrough RLS*. Your increased symptoms might be caused by a new aggravator, and if you can identify and avoid the aggravator, you may be able to reduce the symptoms to a level the medication can treat effectively. Rather than assuming you need to raise your dosage, apply the steps of the Reduction Plan, try several tricks from your BOT, allow your body to adjust, and wait patiently for your current dosage of medicines to work.

5. **The *end of the line* isn't fun.** Many RLSers discard all their old tricks when they start with prescription medicines. They think they are beyond any benefits that could come from using tricks like distraction, massage, or music. They stop looking at aggravators and deficiencies that might be reduced. Then, once they have tried all the drugs and are told there is nothing more the doctor can prescribe to help them, they are devastated. It is much wiser to continue developing your Bag of Tricks, to continue applying the Reduction Plan, and to constantly

be improving your approach to using your BOT, so you never run out of options.

6. *Drug holidays* **may call for using old tricks.** When prescription medications stop working effectively, many doctors will recommend *drug holidays*. During a drug holiday, RLSers go for a period of time without a medicine that has stopped working. Drug holidays give the RLSer's body time to adjust and reduce its tolerance to the drug. During this time, many RLSers suddenly have to rely on self-help tricks they may not have used in months, or even years. As we have learned, many of those tricks require skill and practice if they are to be applied effectively. Once again, it makes sense to use a combination approach, where you keep all your tricks dusted off and in use, so they are there and reliable when needed.

Four categories of drug options

In general, medications used for RLS tend to fall into the four categories described below. I have provided a description of each of the four main categories and a few examples of medicines in each group. I am not recommending any of these, nor saying they will help you with your unique symptoms. As with my examples of other prop tricks, I merely offer the names of these medicines as examples for you to consider. I have tried to use the names I hear most often from RLSers who use them. Some of them are brand names, while others are generic. In some cases, I may refer to a type of medication, rather than a specific medication. The following information is a general overview and a good place to start your research into prescription medications.

1. *Dopaminergic Agents:* This category includes dopamine precursors and dopamine-receptor agonists. Dopamine precursors deliver levodopa to the brain, where it is

converted into dopamine. A commonly used drug in this category is carbidopa/levodopa (Sinemet). If the levodopa were taken alone, it would never make it to the brain. The carbidopa acts like a private taxi service, taking the levodopa right to the edge of the brain and delivering it to do its work.

The other type of dopaminergic drugs are called dopamine-receptor agonists, and include drugs like Permax, Mirapex, and Requip. Be aware that drugs like Sinemet can seem to work miracles at first, but can also lead to *augmentation*. Augmentation is where the RLS symptoms start developing earlier in the day and become more severe than before using the medication. Some of these drugs also result in *rebound*, which means they start losing effectiveness before the end of the dosing period. If this happens, increasing the dosage can actually make things worse. For more information, consult with your doctor.

While the drugs in this category can help reduce RLS symptoms, they can also cause side effects, including insomnia and gastrointestinal problems. Some of these negative side effects will diminish with time. Your doctor may have ideas for counteracting the side effects, making it easier to stick with the drug and enjoy its benefits.

2. *Opioids:* These are known to many of us as *pain killers*. They can be effective with RLS symptoms, even if pain is not a complaint. Use of opioids can cause concern because of their negative side effects (e.g., sleep apnea, addiction). However, with constant vigilance for undesirable effects, many RLS patients are able to effectively use opioids on a daily basis. Examples of drugs in this category might be Codeine, Percocet, Vicodin, and Darvon.

    Opioids are considered to have sedative qualities, which means they can impair your ability to do activities that require alertness. They also have potential physical side effects that may require the adjustment of dosages. The other real problem to RLSers who need this medication is the potential difficulty obtaining a drug that is highly regulated and restricted by law. This is something you want to discuss with your doctor before becoming reliant on a medication that might be difficult to obtain over the long run.

3. *Benzodiazepines:* These drugs work by quieting the central nervous system and are known to many people as tranquilizers or anti-anxiety drugs. They may be useful in promoting sleep and relieving anxiety, even though they don't actually stop RLS symptoms. They are usually used at nighttime, but can cause daytime sleepiness. Examples of benzodiazepines include, Klonopin, Valium, and Xanax. There are other drugs used for inducing sleep that are not benzodiazepines, but are used with a similar purpose (e.g., Ambien).

4. *Anticonvulsants:* This category of drugs seems to be useful for daytime RLS control, especially when there is a complaint of associated pain. These may also have sedative effects (e.g., impairing alertness), along with having several relatively common physical side effects that may be controllable by other methods. Examples of anticonvulsants are Neurontin, Depakote, and Tegretol.

Prescription and intravenous iron treatments

Prescription iron supplements provide more iron than over-the-counter iron products. Excessive doses of iron can also be administered intravenously. Impressive results have been produced in studies where iron was given intravenously, causing a significant rise in ferritin (iron storage) levels. As more is learned of this process and the long-term results, it may become a valuable form of prescription medicine to add to your BOT.

Don't let your prescription drugs deplete you

If you use prescription medications on a regular basis, be sure to question the possible deficiencies that may result. For instance, it is not uncommon for prescription drugs to deplete B-12. This could create a problem, since B-12 deficiencies are suspected to trigger RLS symptoms.

Some drugs can affect your liver or digestive system, requiring you to have constant monitoring. You might want to ask your doctor about using supplements to counteract the depletions or negative effects of drugs on your organs. You want to avoid a scenario where the drugs help until they leave you with a deficiency that triggers worse RLS symptoms.

Keep the big picture in mind

Though we have focused a great deal on relieving RLS symptoms, always remember the big picture: the desire to improve your quality of life. You don't want to achieve RLS symptom relief at the cost of feeling like a zombie 24/7 or being unable to fulfill daily responsibilities to your job or family. It takes time to balance prescription medications, but with good communication, you and your doctor should be able to find the right combination of treatments. Focus on developing good teamwork with your doctor, maintaining a diverse BOT, and achieving symptom relief in the easiest and safest manner.

Is It Worth a Try?

IT IS EASY to lose your better judgment when you are sleep deprived. Exhaustion can make it hard to resist a great sales pitch that promises relief from your Restless Legs Syndrome (RLS) symptoms.

Many new ideas and gadgets look wonderful when you are telling yourself, "I'd do anything to not have these awful urges to move."

With a little knowledge and insight, some gimmicks are relatively transparent. If they claim to cure a long list of problems, red flags should go up quickly. In fact, just the word *cure* or a claim to *cure all*, is definite reason to be skeptical. A long list of testimonials from cured customers is another cause for red flags. Some sales pitches are hard to see coming.

I am often suckered in when I hear, "I just found something that works great for me, and I just had to tell you about it."

It finally dawns on me that I'm into a gimmick when I say I'm not interested and they start accusing me of being the kind of person who loves to suffer. Even when I know I'm being given a polished sales pitch from a multi-level marketing salesperson, I am often left wondering if I just passed up a trick that would have cured me, if I had just tried it.

When in doubt, ask questions

Consider some of the following questions, if you are still tempted to try a new trick, but you keep hearing your inner voice saying, "Watch out!"

1. *Does it sound too good to be true?* Usually, when something sounds too good to be true, it is. Knowing that RLS is different for everyone, what are the chances that the product will work as well as all the testimonials claim? Pay attention to sales pitches claiming better results than seem possible. On the other hand, do not let an overly zealous sales pitch prevent you from recognizing the benefits of an otherwise worthwhile product. The idea might have merit if represented properly. Decide whether there is any chance it will help you, even if it doesn't *cure* your RLS. Determine whether the product has ingredients that make sense to you. If it still looks useful, ask yourself whether you could create the same effect with a simpler or cheaper version.

2. *Can you afford this?* We tend to say, "If it works, I can afford anything."
   Whether it's prescription medicines or alternative supplements and gadgets, the costs can be high and drain your resources over the coming years. Be careful. Aggravating your RLS by creating financial stress could be counterproductive.

3. *Even if it doesn't relieve your RLS, is there a chance it will just feel good and be worth it for the pleasant feelings?* Don't let false claims and bad advertising keep you from enjoying a trick that might bring relief or relaxation. As long as you have realistic expectations, you might enjoy having another prop trick to use.

4. *Is there a chance it will relieve symptoms from other aggravating physical, emotional, or mental conditions*

and indirectly bring you RLS relief? Again, the claim that it will cure your RLS might not hold true, but the product might help with other ailments or symptoms.

5. *Are you really likely to use this gadget or treatment, or will it be one more thing to spend money on that ends up sitting in the closet?* Be honest. We all intend to be disciplined and stick to a plan, but if you know yourself well and know you are more likely to get up and walk than to grab a special gadget and use it, why spend money on it?

6. *Is there research to back up the claims? Where does the research come from? What is the anecdotal evidence? How many people were studied? What variables were controlled?* These are all typical questions pertaining to things that might be scientifically studied. The problem is, many props are useful and worth your time and money, but will never be scientifically tested because they are not worth the time and money of the researchers. You have to use your own best judgment when determining safety, reliability, and wisdom of using the product. When there are studies, learn to analyze them to determine if their results really apply to your needs. If they tested fifty people in a nursing home, their results might be different than what would apply to your eight-year-old who has RLS. Analyze, learn, question, and make up your own mind.

7. *Do you understand how to use the gadget or treatment?* Often, the gadget or treatment can seem ineffective when it is really a problem of the user not following the instructions. With prescription drugs, for example, you wouldn't try one pill and give up. They are usually used according to a prescribed plan of dosing. Ask yourself if there are instructions that go along with this new gadget or treatment. Then follow directions and give it a fair try.

Sometimes the slightest change in use can make a difference in whether a trick is useful. For example, my *rubber band trick*, where you put a therapy band around the ball of your foot and then flex your foot, doesn't work if the band is around the arch of your foot. It's only a difference of a couple of inches, but those couple of inches can prevent a normally effective trick from working.

8. ***Can you use the product safely?*** Are there precautions to take if you use the product? Could the product have negative effects on other ailments or problems? You might need to support your back, use a lower temperature, take less of it, or not do something for as long a time, or as vigorously, because of your extenuating circumstances and health. Remember, if you do not use a trick the way it was designed to be used, it may not work effectively for you.

9. ***Is this product or treatment duplicating something you are already taking?*** For example, if it is an herbal or mineral supplement or nutrient, is it doing the same thing as one of your prescription medications, thereby possibly overdoing a good thing or creating an additional problem?

10. ***Can it interact with anything you are already taking or doing?*** Some self-help tricks can actually work against prescription medications, or vice versa. Make sure your combination of tricks is complementary.

11. ***Are there any long-term or immediate side effects?*** Every trick has potential side effects. A percussion massager can bruise or hurt. Incorrect use of aromatic oils can create problems. Prescription drugs can deplete your system of important vitamins. Remember, if it's working, it's potent, and it may be doing more than you think.

12. ***Do you trust the source?*** I have received many offers for things that people claimed would relieve me, if not cure me, of my RLS symptoms. One offer came from someone who lived on some island in the Pacific. He wanted to send me, free of charge, his island's natural (and very strong) kava kava. I saw some real problems with trusting the person and his foreign product.

Be a little skeptical, but don't lose hope

I can't possibly try all the tricks that cross my path, but sometimes I feel guilty for not giving them a chance. It can sound and feel as though I have given up hope.

I have chided myself, thinking, "Anyone who claims to be so desperate for relief should surely try a new hope or promise."

However, after trying so many things and having their hopes dashed so many times, RLSers begin to be careful, to discriminate, and to doubt. So when I come across something interesting but don't have the time, money, energy, or enough faith in its potential to try it, I just record it in my notebook. I might put it in the Reduce Panic section or the Gather Tricks section, where I list tricks I might try. That way, I am not turning everything down and acting like a pessimistic victim who says, "Nothing will work."

I believe there are more great tricks that can help, but there is no way I can try them all. Though I may not try every trick that comes along, I hope I will always be aware of new discoveries and advances in RLS treatment. The difficulty is in being just skeptical enough to avoid wasting time, emotions, and money, while staying open to the possibilities of valuable new treatments. I never want the day to come when I am afraid to try another trick because I am too discouraged by treatments that didn't fulfill their promises. There's always room for the hope of a new discovery.

MORE REBEL IDEAS
and AMMUNITION

Can Children Be RLS Rebels?

WHEN I FIRST discovered the name "Restless Legs Syndrome" (RLS), the prevailing information said it was a syndrome of middle-aged people, not likely to plague children. As news of RLS spread, it was soon learned that children experience RLS too. It is mind-boggling to think how many wiggly children have been punished or mislabeled for something no one understood.

There are guidelines now for diagnosing RLS in babies. Consequently, there are also doctors treating patients at a very young age. Parents can play an important role in not only alleviating the RLS symptoms in children, but also in training children to become RLS rebels who independently control their RLS survival program into adulthood.

Be a parental rebel

If you have skipped to this chapter without reading about the RLS Rebel Program, I strongly encourage you to read those chapters and become familiar with the steps of the program. Until your children are old enough to learn the program, you will have to be their *rebel advocate*. You can use all the steps of the RLS Rebel Program to help minimize your children's RLS symptoms and help them deal with at-rest activities.

The REDUCTION PLAN

Step 1: Reduce PANIC (*Get educated*)

Find information about diagnosing and treating childhood RLS. The RLS Foundation's free brochure titled "RLS in Children" can be seen at http://www.rls.org or requested by phone (507) 287-6465.

Step 2: Reduce CHAOS (*Analyze symptoms*)

Make notes of when RLS symptoms appear and how your child describes them. Determine whether certain activities create different types of RLS symptoms and require special responses.

Step 3: Reduce SYMPTOMS (*Identify coexisting ailments*)

Determine whether other ailments are triggering your child's RLS symptoms. With your child's input (if possible), decide which symptoms can be handled by walking or distraction and which symptoms need to be treated with other remedies.

Step 4: Reduce DEFICIENCIES (*Adjust supplement*)

Ask your child's doctor to test for ferritin and other deficiencies. Ask the doctor about the safety of using supplements that are commonly recommended for RLSers.

Step 5: Reduce AGGRAVATORS (*Identify triggers*)

Analyze whether certain foods, medicines, activities, or emotions tend to make the child's RLS symptoms worse.

Step 6: Reduce SITUATIONS (*Prioritize needs*)

Identify and avoid (if possible) potential RLS-provoking situations that are not essential to the child's life or happiness.

The BAG of TRICKS APPROACH (BOTA)

Step 1: GATHER YOUR TRICKS (*List all treatment options*). Keep lists of options for RLS treatments. Someday, the child will have a wonderful foundation on which to base treatment choices.

Step 2: PACK YOUR BAGS *(Match treatments with activities)* Organize the tricks according to the activity where they might be used. Include combinations of prop and no-prop tricks.

Step 3: PLAN OF ATTACK *(Your plan for getting through an activity)* Know and record a plan for preventing or responding to RLS in specific situations.

Step 4: RELIEF PLANS *(Your plan to stop symptoms, immediately)* Teach your child to practice *zero tolerance*. If the child is a baby, *zero tolerance* might mean you give the baby a 2:00 A.M. bath or massage, because you know a bath will quickly stop the RLS symptoms. If the child is older, *zero tolerance* might mean you understand when the child needs to get out of bed and walk before going back to bed and trying another Plan of Attack.

Start your child's RLS Rebel Program file system

It is never too early to start a rebel notebook or file system for a child. You can organize records according to the outline of the RLS Rebel Program (above). Record everything you learn, all the techniques you try, and all the aggravators and deficiencies you adjust.

Along with keeping a notebook or file system of your child's personal RLS program, you can teach (by example, if the child is too young to understand) how to apply *zero tolerance*. As early as possible, teach the child to stop an RLS attack the minute it starts. You can also apply techniques like *bully noise* which will help the child learn to use distraction to overpower RLS symptoms.

As your child grows, be sure to share the records you have kept. Use RLS Rebel Program terminology and explain the various steps of the program. Someday, you will give your child the RLS rebel notebook or file system, and it will be a smooth transition into adult RLS survival. Your efforts will encourage and model valuable attitudes of empowerment and determination.

RLS and babies

RLS information has changed since 1998, when I first learned my need to wiggle was called Restless Legs Syndrome. At that time, they suspected it was a condition for middle-aged people. In the following years, they learned it also occurred in children, and, in fact, might be hereditary. The first time I heard a discussion about RLS in babies was at a 2004 Restless Legs Syndrome Foundation national conference. The discussion was about how the diagnosis process had to be slightly different for infants.

With older children and adults, we can ask the four main diagnostic questions: 1) Do you have an irresistible urge to move? 2) Does it happen when you are at-rest or being still? 3) Does it tend to happen more in the evening? 4) Is it relieved by movement or distraction?

Obviously, babies can't answer these questions. In place of questions, we assume RLS might be present if the usual criteria appear to be happening (i.e., irritable movement when at-rest, more prominent at the end of the day, and relieved with movement or distraction). We can also suspect we are seeing RLS in babies when the normal symptoms are accompanied by a family history of RLS, especially in older siblings who fit the normal diagnostic criteria.

Though I do not remember all the sleep habits of my own two children, I remember saying, "I would have had ten more children if mine would have slept through the night."

Obviously, we had some sleep issues. In light of the fact both children (in their late twenties) now say they have RLS, there is a good chance they were experiencing it then, too. When one of my new grandbabies kept giving her parents fits during the night, I was convinced a part of what many of us call colic might very well be symptoms of RLS in babies.

In this chapter, I will offer thoughts and considerations for parents of children dealing with RLS. If you have a child with RLS, I hope some of these ideas will help you deal with their symptoms and help your children grow into RLSers who feel empowered and feel a sense of control over the *RLS bully*.

Treat with sleep

RLS is often described as a sleep disorder, even though many RLSers do not complain of RLS keeping them from sleeping. More accurately, it is a movement disorder. Some people actually use sleep as a way to rid themselves of an RLS attack. Until I was in my forties, my best way to deal with RLS symptoms was to quickly get to sleep. Sometimes that meant a quick power nap, but sometimes it just meant calling it a night and getting to sleep as fast as possible. In those days, *getting to sleep* was not the issue.

Sometimes, extreme tiredness is the real trigger. If your child often complains of leg pains, or other symptoms that you suspect to be RLS, you might encourage the child to take a quick nap or to go to sleep a little earlier, before exhaustion sets in. With children, it might help to view RLS symptoms as a sign that it is time to go to sleep. It might be best to eliminate evening activities that require the child to sit still. Hot baths might help the child feel ready for sleep, but sitting through bedtime stories might aggravate the RLS.

Convey positive outlooks and feelings of empowerment

Our tendency is to feel sorry for children with RLS, especially if we have known the agony of living with RLS symptoms. It is important to remember that children are fortunate if they have parents who understand and know how to respond to

RLS. Many children do not have that benefit. Instead, they are told to sit still, go to sleep, and quit whining. Many of us were told our symptoms were "growing pains." We were led to believe it would all go away when we finished growing. Today's children can find support and encouragement as they learn to survive with RLS.

Your actions and conversations should convey the positive outlook your child can have. Be careful of words you use that might convey a negative outlook. It would not help to refer to symptoms as the *beast of RLS*. Instead, we can refer to the obnoxious *RLS bully*. Many schools now have anti-bullying rules, so it will make sense to children that RLS bullies are not allowed to dominate.

Encourage your child to feel empowered against the ridiculous signals to wiggle. Explain that with time and practice, your child will get better at fighting the *RLS bully*. The last thing you want to convey to a child is that RLS will become more severe with age. There is no proof that symptoms will get worse. If they do increase, an empowered child will have the best chance of successfully dealing with more severe symptoms.

Encourage your child to become an RLS rebel and start fighting back. A good rebel will have pre-planned offensive strategies that will keep most RLS symptoms at bay. It is also important to have a ready defense for times when the *RLS bully* sneaks through the lines. Encourage your child to be ready to fight, with all his tricks lined up and practiced. This is much better than leaving the child feeling helpless and victimized by the irresistible urges to move.

Listen carefully to descriptions of symptoms

It is difficult for RLSers to describe RLS symptoms. Make sure your child is describing RLS symptoms and not muscle cramps or other problems that might need a different type of attention. Is the child feeling irresistible urges to move or is he feeling pain? Is there a chance something else is wrong?

When you ask your child to describe the feelings, you might hear anything from "my legs ache" to comments about pain, itching, bugs crawling, or cramping. If the child points to a spot and touches it, there is a chance he is pointing to a pain, rather than an RLS urge. RLSers tend to show an *area* where the feelings occur. If the child waves a hand over an area and seems frustrated at not being able to show you exactly where the feeling is, it would be typical of an RLSer.

Determine whether the symptoms occur more when your child is at-rest or late in the day, and whether the symptoms are relieved by movement or distraction. Help the child describe when the feelings are likely to occur (e.g., during what activities and at what time of day). Ask the child what tricks work to alleviate the feelings. All of these are important clues for you to use, and important notes to add to your child's notebook. Asking the child for in-depth descriptions and making notes of the answers will reassure the child you are taking him seriously.

If you are still not sure the child is describing RLS symptoms, you may have to rely on family history. If siblings or parents have RLS, there is a good chance the child is describing RLS symptoms. For a young child with RLS, it might be helpful and even therapeutic to draw a picture of RLS. The first pictures might be of how RLS symptoms feel, or they might be pictures of the child's version of the *RLS bully*. Later, pictures might show the child fighting the *RLS bully*. It would be interesting to note whether the size of the *RLS bully* changes over time in relation to the size of the child. Do the pictures show the child is beginning to feel empowered against RLS symptoms? It may be difficult for a small child to describe abstract urges to wiggle, but the child's drawings may help you understanding exactly what frustrations are being felt.

Once you and your child get a better idea of how the RLS symptoms are manifesting themselves, your child will feel less like a helpless victim. A big part of being ready to deal with RLS symptoms is knowing what to expect. Remember, if you can describe RLS, you can predict it, and if you can predict it, you can be ready to treat it successfully.

Teach *zero tolerance*

When you are teaching your child to deal with RLS, it might be one of the few times you will encourage intolerance. The child needs to understand that RLS symptoms get worse when they are ignored. When sitting still is not possible, quick action is needed to stop the RLS symptoms immediately. The child still needs to behave, but might be allowed special privileges (e.g., getting up, walking, stretching). The faster a planned response to stop the RLS symptoms is applied, the better.

Emphasize no-prop tricks

In an earlier chapter, I discussed some helpful no-prop tricks. These are the best tricks for children to use, because they will not have to remember to have a special prop with them. If they can remember to walk, stretch, or find a mental distraction that will instantly stop the RLS symptoms, they will become confident RLS rebels. The techniques of brushing might be one of their better tricks. You might want to teach them to pretend they have imaginary *RLS rubbing cream* in their hand and can rub it wherever they feel the urges. Early on, they can learn to use this and other instant and powerful responses to deal with obnoxious RLS symptoms.

Talk with teachers

Children with RLS have long been considered behavioral problems in school. (I don't like to think about how many children with RLS have been told, "Sit still!") Encourage good communication between RLS children and their teachers. Educate teachers with articles, books, or Internet websites that describe RLS. Rather than making excuses for your child or asking for special treatment, strive for cooperation and understanding. A desk at the side of a classroom might allow a child to stand and stretch without disturbing others. Children might have more luck sitting still during a movie, lecture, or long exam, if they know it's okay to take a quick walk in the hallway or to stand and stretch at the back wall.

An informed teacher will learn to spot the wiggly child and ask the child to run a short errand so the child can stretch, rather than reprimanding the child for not sitting still. The child and teacher might even develop a hand signal or a code word to signal the need for an RLS break. A little understanding will go a long way toward preventing and responding to RLS in the classroom.

Teach responsibility and politeness

These days, people with disabilities have many rights and privileges. I believe a certain amount of responsibility and good manners is called for when enjoying those special privileges. A child who expects permission to stand by the wall when RLS symptoms occur during class must learn to do this quietly and with the least possible distraction to others. The child should also learn when it is appropriate to wait until there will be the least interruption to the teacher or class. An RLSer's disability and special needs should not be an excuse for rudeness or inconsideration for others. Teachers need to see the special requests of RLS children as easy solutions to otherwise difficult classroom issues. You will find teachers much more cooperative if special needs can be addressed with a minimal amount of distraction to others.

Teach children about *bully noise* and mental distraction tricks

Most children will love the idea of using music to get to sleep. With the help of their parents, children can learn to select "music to go to sleep by." They can have fun choosing music that they are willing to listen to night after night as they hypnotize themselves to sleep.

Children can also learn to rely on suckers, popcorn, peanuts, or raisins for getting through car trips and movies. Help them understand that an empty or bored mind is a perfect attraction for the *RLS bully*. They can learn to use music and food as a way to create movement or mental activity.

Teach children to pack and use their BOT

A child who needs reading glasses must remember to always take them to school. A child who needs medicines must coordinate with the school nurse to have medicines administered on schedule. A child who deals with RLS symptoms during a movie, at a sleepover, or on a field trip, must have a Bag of Tricks (BOT) ready when needed.

Encourage children to plan ahead and not be caught unprepared when the *RLS bully* attacks. It should eventually become the child's responsibility to request an aisle seat, wear comfortable clothing, or take along a sucker (making sure the teacher or supervisor approves its use). At a sleepover, a child might learn to strategically place his sleeping bag near the door to avoid feeling trapped or cut off from the escape route.

Before a child begins an RLS-provoking activity, a parent can help by asking if the child has packed a BOT with reliable prop tricks. This would also be a good time to remind a child to use no-prop tricks (e.g., walking, distraction). Just as a squadron leader might review plans for a mission, a parent and child can review a practical Plan of Attack and Relief Plan to use for the upcoming activity.

Pre-think your responses

Our first tendency is to feel sorry for children with RLS, but we need to remember how resilient children can be, especially when they have the support of understanding families. If we are RLSers ourselves, we do not want to risk passing our feelings of frustration on to our children. To avoid this, anticipate your child's complaints and have planned responses, so you are not misguided by your frustrations or sympathy.

If you are with a child who is experiencing an RLS attack, it is best if you are ready with helpful comments or questions.

If the child is old enough to have a BOT, you can simply ask, "What is the best thing for you to do when this happens? What is your Plan of Attack or Relief Plan?"

If the child is too young to manage a BOT, it will be up to you to quickly employ a Plan of Attack that you have previously developed for the child.

You can ask, "Does it help to rub your legs or press them to the floor like you are walking? Would it help to suck on a sucker while you watch television?"

By doing this, you will be leaving the responsibility with your child and be helping him feel empowered and in control. Avoid beginning your sentence with the word "why." When you ask, "Why don't you suck on a sucker?" it is easy for the child to feel stupid for not thinking of it before you suggested it.

While RLS symptoms are present, it is time to rely on strategies already in place.

If the child is traveling in a car and complains of crazy leg feelings, you can be ready with helpful questions, such as, "Would it help to rub it out with imaginary *RLS rubbing cream?*" Or you might ask, "Do you think the pretend-walking trick would help?"

If a young child is supposed to be sleeping, but wanders into the living room and says, "My legs hurt. I can't sleep," be ready with responses that fit a first Relief Plan. After a glass of water and a quick hug and kiss, encourage the child to go back to sleep and practice the Plan of Attack for getting to sleep. The plan might be to "Wiggle, take two deep breaths, count to fifty, and recite a poem in your head or listen to music."

If the child wanders in again, you can be ready to respond with a more involved Relief Plan that might include stretching, talking, a massage, or an undesirable exercise, like running up and down the stairs ten times. Remember, Relief Plan tricks are movement and mental distraction exercises, not punishment. They do not need to be unpleasant things to do, but neither should they be terribly exciting or rewarding.

If the child wanders in a third time, you can apply a third Relief Plan, which might include a hot bath or a task such as cleaning the child's room. Help the child understand that cleaning a bedroom fulfills the goal of using physical movement and mental distraction to combat RLS symptoms. Once the movement or distraction calms the RLS urges, the child can get back to bed and use a Plan of Attack to get to sleep.

When you pre-think your comments, you are helping your child learn routine responses to RLS symptoms. Eventually, the child will independently use the responses you have modeled.

When the child needs to wiggle, he will hear you asking, "What works for you when this happens?"

Until the child is ready to take responsibility, you can be ready with logical, reasonable, and helpful responses, rather than frustrated pleas for the child to just be still.

Convey happiness and support

In my observation, children with disabilities are more likely to be happy if they have been taught to handle their problems as inconspicuously and independently as possible. I have seen children with more illness and disability than I can imagine anyone dealing with, yet they acted as though they were not only normal, but fortunate and blessed. This is the attitude we need to convey to children with RLS.

RLS can be an enormous burden if you are not prepared to deal with the symptoms. However, if you are prepared, and you are supported by your loved ones, you can survive and even thrive with RLS. Today's RLS children are more fortunate than those in the past, who were thought to have behavior problems or who feared they might become ten feet tall if their "growing pains" didn't hurry up and stop.

In a later chapter, I will cover how to be a good supporter of someone with RLS. I will describe the most valuable thing any supporter can provide. Be sure to take a look at that chapter as you consider other ways you might help a child with RLS.

To Our RLS Healthcare Providers

IDEALLY, HEALTHCARE PROVIDERS will read all of *The RLS Rebel's Survival Guide,* but if time is limited, the following information will give healthcare providers a preliminary understanding of the RLS Rebel Program and will facilitate better communication between medical professionals and their Restless Legs Syndrome (RLS) patients.

The RLS Rebel's Survival Guide

The following information comes from the book, *Restless Legs Syndrome: The RLS Rebel's Survival Guide,* by Jill Gunzel, BEd, MEd, and RLSer for more than forty-five years. The book describes the RLS Rebel Program, an outline which helps RLSers (patients with RLS) organize their fight against RLS and achieve maximize results from a combination of treatments. When treatments include prescription drugs, the RLS Rebel Program is the ultimate guide for a complementary medicine approach to RLS.

The RLS Rebel Program begins with six steps of the Reduction Plan. By addressing the six steps, RLSers reduce variables that trigger out-of-control RLS symptoms. By reducing symptoms, treatments will become more effective. In the second part of the RLS Rebel Program, the RLSer is encouraged to develop a Bag of Tricks Approach (BOTA): a combination of treatments systematically applied to at-rest activities. The book also explains how the RLS Rebel Program can be used when treating children with RLS, helping RLSers travel comfortably, and dealing with surgery and other special situations that can provoke increased symptoms.

The RLSer is encouraged to use the outline of the RLS Rebel Program to set up a notebook or file system. By repeatedly visiting sections of the outline, the RLSer will monitor aggravating variables, maintain an effective combination of treatments, and continually minimize the frequency and severity of RLS symptoms. The outline can easily be used to guide communications between the doctor and RLS patient.

Your RLS rebel patient

RLS patients who use *The RLS Rebel's Survival Guide* are encouraged to be active participants in their health care. They recognize the absence of an easy fix for RLS and are committed to the hard work of learning to survive with a certain degree of RLS symptoms. They value the benefits of working as a team with a medical professional. As a team, you and your RLS rebel patient can cover all the bases, use the most effective diagnostic methods, and employ the safest and most effective combinations of tricks. The following points are offered to help you support your RLS rebel patient.

1. **New RLS information:** Until 2005, I recommended every RLSer and medical professional treating RLS read *Sleep Thief,* by Virginia Wilson. This book documents research, medical opinions, and reports from RLSers prior to 1996. It is still an excellent compilation of medical and lay information on RLS. It also provides an excellent history of various RLS events, including the formation of the Restless Legs Syndrome Foundation.

   In 2005, coinciding with the first FDA approval of an RLS medicine, advertising became widespread and several books were authored by well-respected doctors and authorities in the RLS field. The books (including

The RLS Rebel's Survival Guide) are due for publication in 2006. Some were directed to medical professionals, while others were directed to RLSers.

A free medical bulletin is available online from the national RLS Foundation. In addition, they have publications on special situations (e.g., *Pregnancy and RLS, Surgery and RLS, Children and RLS*). For further information, call the RLS Foundation (507-287-6465) or view their educational publications and downloads at http://www.rls.org.

2. **Sensory motor vs. psychological:** Studies have shown a lack of iron in the brain cells of people who had RLS compared with people who did not have RLS. The discovery of this physical difference helps to establish RLS as a sensory motor disorder, rather than a psychological condition. Because the brain cells are only iron deficient and not damaged, there is great hope for successful treatment of the disorder. The relationship between these iron deficient brain cells and dopamine synthesis makes dopamine management an interesting consideration for treatment.

3. **Ferritin levels:** Management of serum ferritin levels is critical to RLS treatment. Make sure your RLSer has a level of 50ng/ml or more, even though "normal" might be as low as 10ng/ml. Studies have shown a marked decrease of RLS symptoms when serum ferritin levels are raised to at least 50ng/ml.

4. **Primary vs. secondary RLS:** An understanding of the differences between *primary RLS* and *secondary RLS* can affect the way you treat your RLS patient. Primary RLS is associated with childhood onset, a family history of RLS, and no apparent triggering condition or ailment. Secondary RLS is associated with the presence of a condition that may have triggered the start of RLS symp-

toms (e.g., end stage renal disease, back injury, surgery, pregnancy). As in the case of pregnancy, secondary RLS can occur in a person who otherwise would not be prone to RLS symptoms.

If you are treating a patient with no other history of RLS and you suspect a case of secondary RLS, consider treating the RLS indirectly by first addressing the triggering ailment or condition. Keep in mind that a person with primary RLS can experience a sudden increase in severity of symptoms, caused by an overlapping case of secondary RLS. An excellent example of this would be when pregnancy or a new medication triggers secondary RLS. The person might have been effectively handling primary RLS symptoms since childhood and suddenly experience increased symptoms. Instead of assuming the RLS is worsening with age, help the patient see how pregnancy, surgery, or a new medication can trigger a temporary and treatable case of secondary RLS.

5. **Diagnosis:** There is no clinical test for RLS. However, the syndrome can be diagnosed fairly accurately by answering four questions: 1) Does the patient experience irresistible urges to move? 2) Do symptoms occur when the patient is at rest? 3) Are symptoms more likely to occur in the evening? 4) Are symptoms relieved by movement or distraction?

Observe how your patient describes the RLS sensations. Most RLSers will not point to or actually touch a specific spot. They are more likely to wave their hands about six inches over their legs or arms, indicating the general area where RLS sensations tend to occur. If an RLS patient touches a spot, and says, "I feel it right there," investigate the possibility of another ailment (e.g., arthritis, peripheral neuropathy, sciatica).

6. **Reduce the *beast of RLS*:** When RLS symptoms rage out of control, RLSers sometime refer to them as the *beast of RLS*. The Reduction Plan (Part I of the RLS Rebel Program), helps the RLSer address six areas that can affect the severity and frequency of RLS symptoms. By addressing these six areas, the RLSer can reduce the *beast of RLS* to mere bully size. Conventional and alternative treatments will be more effective against the *RLS bully* than against the *beast of RLS*. As RLS rebel patients address the six areas of the Reduction Plan, they will need your help in testing for conflicting ailments, analyzing and managing deficiencies, and sorting through the latest RLS studies and information.

7. **Agree on treatment priorities:** RLS symptoms lead to many simultaneous complaints.

   An RLSer might report all of the following complaints: "I'm exhausted. I can't sit still. I have a terrible time trying to get to sleep. When I do sleep, I wake several times during the night and can't get back to sleep. I have pain. I'm depressed. I'm anxious. I can't get my work done on the job because I can't sit still."

   Discuss treatment priorities with your RLS patient. Some RLSers can handle their daytime RLS symptoms, but need help getting to sleep. Other RLSers can get to sleep, but need help sitting still during the day. Be aware that some of the most commonly prescribed medications for RLS will fix one need while making another situation worse (e.g., calming the RLS symptoms but causing insomnia).

   Make sure your patient understands what results to expect from each medication. Many RLSers end up with more than one medication for treating RLS. The patient may not realize which medicine is meant to help induce sleep and which is meant to help him sit still during the day. If the intended results of the various medicines are not understood, the RLSer is likely to report the medicine was not effective, when in fact, the medicine may have worked exactly as intended.

8. **Avoid dosage confusion:** Because RLSers tend to be tired and frustrated, they have to be extra careful to take correct dosages of medications. At 3:00 A.M., it is easy to be confused about what has been taken and what is still okay to use. Many RLSers are prescribed *drug cocktails* (combinations of medications) and find it a real management challenge to remember what to take, in which combinations, with or without food, or what dosage is appropriate.

   A common source of dosage confusion occurs if dosages are changed while the patient still has medicine in a container labeled with the original prescription dose. Dosage adjustments should be put in writing and placed by the original bottle. Some patients find it helpful to tape a revised dosage label over the old one.

   Dosage confusion can also be avoided by encouraging RLS patients to keep an up-to-date chart of amounts and times when medication should be taken. If patients bring their medication charts to office visits, you can make changes on their charts, sending them home with the latest prescribed dosages. The chart should also provide symbols or notations that tell the patient whether a medication is to be taken all the time or on an *as-needed* basis. Some patients like the liberty to adjust their own dosages, as needed. If this is okay with you, notations can be made on the patient's medication chart, stipulating limitations or guidelines for safe changes in dosages.

9. **Check aggravators before raising the dose:** If an RLSer is complaining of *breakthrough attacks*, despite continued use of a previously effective medicine, do not be in a hurry to raise the dose. First, encourage your patient to

review the six steps of the Reduction Plan. By reviewing the steps of the Reduction Plan, you and your patient might discover new deficiencies (Step 4), new aggravators (Step 5), or new ailments and symptoms (Step 3) affecting the severity of the RLS. The current medication may still be effective, once the aggravating variables are addressed. RLS symptoms can be aggravated by lifestyle changes, stressful events, new ailments, or altered diet.

When an RLSer says his symptoms suddenly got worse, be sure to ask, "What was happening about the time it got worse?"

It is amazing how many times increased symptoms can be triggered by something like divorce, allergies, surgery, back injury, or use of medications (e.g., antihistamines, antidepressants).

Avoid insinuating RLS is *all in the patient's head*, or *just stress*. The cause of RLS is far more elusive than that. Nevertheless, there are many triggers that can be easily adjusted or eliminated, without a need to change medications or treatments.

10. **Rebound, augmentation, and drug holidays:** Some medicines are very effective in low dosages, but can aggravate RLS symptoms when dosages are raised. Sinemet is a prime example. A little of it may seem to work miracles, but too high a dose can actually increase RLS symptoms. If a patient claims a medicine is not working for as long a period as before (rebound), or RLS symptoms are starting earlier than before (augmentation), be suspicious of the medication and be prepared to start juggling and adjusting.

   It is common for RLS symptoms to increase after a medicine has been used for an extended period. Many doctors advise *drug holidays*, finding that a break from a previously effective medicine will make the medicine useful again. This practice also helps maintain the effectiveness of lower dosages. During drug holidays, patients should be reminded to rely on other prescription treatments or self-help methods.

RLS Rebel Program tips

You and your patient can use the RLS Rebel Program as a valuable tool of communication and a well-organized approach to RLS treatment. The following tips will give you a quick introduction and springboard for using the RLS Rebel Program while treating your RLS rebel patient.

1. **Think complementary, not alternative.** The RLS Rebel Program is not an alternative program. It is an organizational approach to minimizing RLS symptoms and managing combinations of treatments. Prescription medications are just one of many possible tricks (treatments) in an RLSer's bag of tricks (BOT). For many reasons, RLSers should never rely on just one treatment.

2. **Use the RLS Rebel Program terminology.** The following terminology was coined for unique application to the RLS Rebel Program:

   An RLSer is a person who experiences RLS symptoms. The nickname was developed as an attempt to avoid the negative implications of labels, like *RLS sufferer* or *RLS victim.*

   RLS rebel is a nickname for anyone who recognizes the absence of an easy RLS fix and commits to the hard work of applying the RLS Rebel Program. An RLS rebel can be a family member, friend, or even a healthcare provider.

   Tricks are treatments used to prevent or respond to RLS symptoms. Just like magic tricks, RLS treatments do not always work. When they do work, they often give the illusion of having cured RLS, but they have brought only temporary relief. A trick can be a prescription medication, alternative treatment, or self-help method. The term *tricks* reminds RLSers to have realistic expectations for all RLS treatments.

No-prop tricks are treatments that do not require any material prop. These tricks include walking, self-massage, concentration, and distraction.

Prop tricks are treatments which require a material prop. These tricks include the use of medications, herbal teas, suckers, therapy bands, and music.

Zero tolerance is an attitude of intolerance for RLS symptoms. The longer an RLS attack continues, the harder it is to stop. If a treatment fails to quickly stop RLS symptoms, the RLSer should use any trick known to work immediately, even if it means stopping the current at-rest activity. Once the obnoxious feelings subside, the activity can be resumed and the original tricks can be used, or relied on, again. Encourage your RLS patients to apply *zero tolerance*, even if all they do is walk.

Bully noise is brain activity that overpowers the urges to wiggle. RLS attacks tend to occur when the mind and body are at rest. An active or noisy mind can be a useful RLS trick. Similar to the practice of using white noise, *bully noise* uses one noise to drown out another. It is based on playground experiences that taught us we could block out the sounds of a bully by sticking our fingers in our ears and yelling louder than our tormentor. If RLSers can view RLS symptoms as a bully and find ways to keep their brain activity busier than the bully's silly taunts to wiggle, they can overpower the urge to move.

3. **Avoid linear approaches.** The RLS Rebel Program advocates a flexible approach to symptom management, combining prescription medications, self-help methods, and lifestyle changes, at any stage where they are effective. Conventional medicine tends to use a linear

approach. Mild to moderate RLS symptoms are treated with self-help methods and lifestyle changes, while prescription medications are reserved as the sole treatment in severe cases.

The problem with a linear approach can be seen at both ends of the spectrum. A person with mild RLS may need prescription medicines to treat temporary bouts of sleep deprivation, special travel situations, or increased symptoms due to changes in lifestyle or health. The option of using medications can build confidence in the RLSer, by providing a powerful and effective treatment when needed. Short-term use of a prescription medicine can also help a newly-diagnosed RLSer quickly catch up on sleep, experience a sharp decrease in RLS symptoms, and reduce anxiety and panic.

At the other end of the severity scale, a person with severe RLS needs to continue using self-help methods and lifestyle changes so medications can be the most effective. If your patient develops a tolerance to a medication, he can rely on a combination of other tricks while taking a *drug holiday*. If the RLSer forgets to pack his medication or fails to get a prescription refilled in time, he can still use effective self-help tricks while waiting to get more medication. If RLSers give up on self-help methods and rely strictly on medications, they will have little choice but to keep trying new medications or raising dosages if their current treatments stop working. When RLSers with severe symptoms rely solely on medications, it is not uncommon for them to run out of options. These are just a few reasons it is important to not only consider a combination of treatments for all stages of RLS, but also to be sure to consider all treatments for all levels of RLS.

4. **Use the RLS Rebel Program Outline.** It can be extremely hard for an exhausted and frustrated RLSer to present

concise feedback to aid you in prescribing treatments. The RLS Rebel Program Outline can be a guide for communicating, clearly and quickly, with RLS patients. A brief review of the steps in the outline will help both you and your patient cover important areas of RLS treatment.

Hopefully, your RLS rebel patient will keep a notebook (organized according to the RLS Rebel Program Outline) in which he will monitor all the steps of the Reduction Plan. The notebook will also be a record of the RLSer's Bag of Tricks Approach (BOTA). The RLSer can also use the notebook to store new information, ideas for new treatments, and questions for the next office visit.

The RLS Rebel Program Outline is presented below. Please refer to the survival guide for detailed information on each part of the outline. By asking some of the questions presented below, you can use the outline to effectively communicate with and treat your RLS patient.

The REDUCTION PLAN

Step 1: Reduce PANIC *(Get educated)*: "Have you come across any new RLS information since we last met?"

Step 2: Reduce CHAOS *(Analyze symptoms)*: "Have you noticed any changes or anything new about the predictability or behavior of your symptoms?"

Step 3: Reduce SYMPTOMS *(Identify coexisting ailments)*: "Have you developed any new symptoms? Are we successfully treating your priority symptoms? Are coexisting ailments aggravating RLS symptoms?"

Step 4: Reduce DEFICIENCIES *(Adjust supplements and diet)*: "What changes have you made to your supplement regime and diet? Have the changes made a difference?"

Step 5: Reduce AGGRAVATORS *(Identify and avoid triggers)*: "Have you identified new aggravators or noticed improvement from avoiding previously identified aggravators?"

Step 6: Reduce SITUATION *(Prioritize needs)*: "What activities are you still avoiding in an effort to minimize your daily RLS symptoms? Are you ready to begin treating for those activities? Are there new activities provoking your RLS that need our attention?"

The BAG OF TRICKS APPROACH (BOTA)

Step 1: GATHER YOUR TRICKS *(List all treatment options)*: "Have you found any new tricks?"

Step 2: PACK YOUR BAGS *(Match treatments with activities)*: "Have the prescription medicines produced the results you were expecting? Have you found other tricks that work well with the medication? Which activities are still provoking enough RLS to prevent you from enjoying the activity?"

Step 3: PLAN OF ATTACK *(Your plan to get through an activity)*: "What is your strategy for getting through your priority activities (e.g., your routine for getting to sleep quickly)?"

Step 4: RELIEF PLANS *(Your plan to stop symptoms immediately)*: "If initial treatments fail, what is your fall-back plan to immediately stop the RLS symptoms?"

Teamwork creates the ultimate in complementary medicine

Even if your RLS patient is not familiar with the RLS Rebel Program, you can present the program's outline as your treatment guide. Explain how the sections of the outline will be used to cover important concerns during RLS treatment. You could go so far as to present the patient with a notebook and encourage him to keep all RLS information, organized according to the RLS Rebel Program Outline.

If your RLS patient follows the RLS Rebel Program Outline and keeps good records, your conversations will be shorter and more productive. The patient will be doing everything possible to get the best results from the treatment protocols you prescribe. When you and your patient use the RLS Rebel Program, you will have a well-organized and effective complementary medicine approach to RLS.

Do's and Don'ts for Dealing with Your Doctor

MANY RLSERS QUESTION whether they should stay with their current doctor or find a new one who specializes in Restless Legs Syndrome (RLS) treatments. If you can find an RLS specialist in your area, it might be best to try that doctor first. However, it is possible you will be just as well off with any doctor you feel is open-minded, eager to learn about RLS, and willing to work as a team. Just as there is not one treatment that works for everyone, there is not one type of doctor that is best. RLS specialists use different drugs and treatment plans, according to their preferences and the patients' needs. The important thing is to find a *special doctor*, rather than a *specialist*.

In many instances, an RLSer's primary care doctor can quickly come up to speed on RLS information. When this happens, the RLSer enjoys the added benefit of being cared for by someone who is already familiar with his health and with whom a good working relationship has already been established. Here are some do's and don'ts for ensuring the best results from the medical professional you turn to for treating your RLS.

1. **DO organize.** Use the RLS Rebel Program to organize your thoughts, needs, questions, and experiences. With everything organized and accessible in the notebook, you can share this information quickly and concisely,

keeping your doctor's interest and keeping the two of you working as a team.

2. **DON'T relinquish responsibility.** Do not turn over all responsibility to your doctor. Stay in charge of your own RLS program. Work toward teamwork, but remember that you are the one who will make all the final decisions.

3. **DO share information.** Offer to share information with your doctor—and I mean *offer*, not *push*. Make sure your doctor is open to receiving information. You can ask the Restless Legs Syndrome Foundation to send professional medical information to your doctor or you can print out website information. The last thing you want to do is give your doctor the opinion you know more, or that your doctor is inadequately educated on the topic. As a team, you can gather and present information while asking your doctor to help interpret and implement ideas. To make this exchange possible, mutual respect has to be carefully maintained.

4. **DON'T "dump on the doc."** Avoid the urge to dump a long list of complaints on your doctor and expect them to be addressed all at once. Instead, prioritize your needs. What do you want to work on first? Maybe you can handle the daytime RLS by walking or keeping busy, but you need help getting to sleep at night, or maybe you want to stay alert while driving, but need to get rid of the urges before you panic and are tempted to jump out of a moving car.

5. **DO keep detailed records.** Use your RLS rebel notebook to keep detailed records, including brands of supplements, dosages of prescription medications, treatment plans, and side effects of treatments. If you decide to re-try an old trick, it will help to have the details of that treatment. If you find information on a new trick you

can't try immediately, detailed notes about the trick will help when the time comes to give the new idea a try.

6. **DON'T jump straight to prescription medications.** First develop a relationship with your doctor, allow time to obtain tests results (e.g. ferritin levels), work on eliminating aggravators, and treat coexisting ailments that might be triggering RLS symptoms. When it comes time for trying medications, you want to be dealing with as few other triggers and aggravators as possible. You will also want to allow time for your doctor to become familiar with the latest RLS information and with the problems you are having with RLS symptoms.

7. **DO check your ferritin.** Be sure your doctor understands *normal* is not a good enough result. You need to be sure your ferritin is 50ng/ml or more. Also ask your doctor about checking for B-12 levels and other possible deficiencies.

8. **DON'T take medicine you don't understand.** Learn what each drug should accomplish. Know its side effects, when to consider the side effects excessive, and when the medicine might interact with other medicines or supplements you are using. Also tell your doctor whether you prefer a medicine you have to use all the time or one you can take *as needed* (PRN).

9. **DO one thing at a time.** Doing one thing at a time means you might add a medicine, remove a medicine, or change the way you are taking a medication. If your doctor hands you a new prescription and also changes the dose of a drug you are already using, that would be two changes at once. Ask if you can change one thing at a time and find out which change to make first. By changing things slowly, you and your doctor can get a better picture of how things are working.

10. **DON'T stand for poor communication.** Find a way to develop a responsible, professional dialogue with your medical team. Obviously, you and your doctor do not have hours to spend talking. Find ways to be concise and get right to the point. Make it easy for someone to respond. Try using brief emails or sending a FAX. If you do this, be specific. State the purpose and critical background information for the correspondence. List your questions (as few as possible). Tell the person how to respond (e.g., by phone, FAX, email). Some doctors may add extra charges for communications by FAX or email. Ask about your doctor's policy and ask about the best way to communicate between visits.

11. **DO stick to the prescription you are given.** Unless your doctor adjusts your original dose, stick with the dosages on the prescription label. Avoid taking too much medicine when in a panic or overwhelmed by RLS symptoms. When in doubt, write down what you take and when you took it. Just as important, do not stop taking a medicine unless you know it is safe to go *cold turkey*. Some medicines have to be changed or discontinued slowly. Just because a small amount worked well, that does not mean more will work better. In fact, with RLS, more of some medicines can make your RLS symptoms worse. If you want the liberty to adjust your medicine as needed, ask your doctor if it is advisable and whether there are limits or safety precautions to making those adjustments.

12. **DON'T assume OTCs are harmless.** Just because something does not require a prescription does not mean it cannot harm you. Herbals, over-the-counter medicines (OTCs), supplements, and homeopathic drugs are potentially harmful. If they are worth the money, they must be effective. If they are effective, they are potent, and potentially dangerous. Tell your doctor what you

are using. Your self-help treatments can affect the treatments your doctor prescribes.

13. **DO keep a list of medications and treatments.** In your RLS rebel notebook, keep an updated list of your medications and treatments. At your next appointment, give the doctor a copy of that list. If the doctor changes a dosage or method of taking a drug, be sure the changes are noted in your notebook and on the doctor's copy of the list you supplied. When you get home, put a copy of the changed list of medications near your medicines. You may want to make changes on the prescription bottle by taping a small note to the bottle so the directions on the bottle will match what you are currently taking.

Sleep Tips

MANY RLSERS REPORT early experiences with Restless Legs Syndrome (RLS) in which they were able to get rid of RLS symptoms by taking a power nap or going straight to bed. Eventually, however, most RLSers say their symptoms interfere with their ability to get to sleep. By the time a person realizes RLS has caused a sleep disorder, bedtime routines and sleep habits may be scrambled or non-existent.

Most of us grow up with little thought to how we go to sleep or stay asleep. When an illness or sleep disorder develops, we must analyze a process which previously happened instinctively. Suddenly, we question what position to lie in, the sounds we hear in the room, temperature, thoughts, and schedules. What was once a natural, almost thoughtless activity becomes an intricate balance of mind, body, and emotions.

The vicious cycle of RLS and sleep deprivation

A vicious cycle occurs when RLS and sleep deprivation appear together. Tiredness, coupled with the fear of not being able to get to sleep and the added problem of RLS symptoms, can become a vicious cycle. RLS symptoms cause restlessness. Restlessness leads to multiple wake ups. Multiple wake ups lead to poor sleep quality. Poor sleep quality leads to sleep deprivation. And finally, lack of quality sleep leads to aggravated RLS symptoms. The cycle goes on, with each part of it perpetuating the next.

Since we don't know where this cycle begins, it is hard to know what part of the problem to address first. Our best bet is to hit it from several angles. We can apply the RLS Rebel Program to the RLS symptoms. We can learn about good sleep hygiene and apply those tips to our bedtime routine. We can analyze daily activities that might affect our sleep and we can change our thought patterns to ones that guide us to better sleep. Medicines can assist us in breaking the cycle, but care needs to be taken to be sure we do not avoid dealing with problems or aggravators that need attention and repair.

Learn more about sleep and sleep deprivation

Sleep deprivation can cause serious physical and emotional problems. The complexity and seriousness of sleep issues has led to the availability of many wonderful books and websites dealing with sleep and sleep habits. I encourage you to do research and find information to help you understand how to develop good sleep habits and achieve quality sleep.

In addition to researching information on sleep, be sure to research your own mental and physical condition. Since physical and emotional problems can affect sleep, I encourage you to determine whether other ailments or emotional issues are interfering with your sleep. Sleep apnea and Periodic Limb Movement Disorder (PLMD) can be diagnosed in a sleep study. If you have these conditions, it would probably help to treat them, too.

The RLS Rebel Program is the place to start when addressing your sleep issues. Using the Reduction Plan and the Bag of Tricks Approach (BOTA) will help you organize all the variables that might affect your ability to get to sleep and your sleep quality. The following RLS-related sleep tips should help you achieve success in getting to sleep, despite RLS symptoms.

Consider how daytime activities affect your sleep

Many RLSers have had to adjust their exercise plans to minimize RLS symptoms. Some find exercise helps reduce RLS symptoms, while others find it is detrimental, especially when it is done too close to bedtime. Experiment and figure out what is best for you.

Though stressful lifestyles can affect an RLSer's sleep, being busy is not necessarily a problem. Sometimes lack of activity can create stress and anxiety that trigger RLS symptoms. I find my worst times are before I start a project. Not knowing what awaits me in a pile of bills is a sure-fire trigger to RLS symptoms. Once I am in the middle of a project, with a full day of multi-tasking and decision making, I am less likely to have problems with RLS symptoms.

"To nap, or not to nap?" That is the question for many. If tiredness is a trigger for your RLS, it may help to take naps. But, if *getting to sleep* is your big problem, you certainly do not want daytime naps to take the edge off your need for sleep. It is possible you will do well with naps, if you take them early in the day. There is no right answer for everyone. Experiment with what napping habits are best for you.

Do foods or supplements affect your sleep?

How much you eat may have as much or more influence on RLS symptoms than *what* you eat. For many RLSers, overeating at Thanksgiving dinner can trigger an RLS attack faster than any other meal of the year. I can eat a big meal at a restaurant that is only a mile from our house and the ride home can bring on excruciating RLS symptoms. I have often found myself thinking I would rather just walk home. Perhaps a short walk before driving home would help the situation. I certainly would not want to go straight to bed after a big meal.

While doing research on nutrition and sleep, I found a list of foods thought to affect quality of sleep. The foods that were thought to work against sleep were described as being high in *tyramine* (said to increase norepinephrine, a brain stimulant). These foods included bacon, cheese, chocolate, eggplant, ham, potatoes, sauerkraut, sugar, sausage, spinach, tomatoes, and wine. The foods thought to promote sleep were high in *tryptophan*. These included, bananas, turkey, figs, dates, yogurt, milk, tuna, and whole grain crackers. I am not recommending these foods, nor am I recommending the supplements of tyramine or tryptophan. I am merely suggesting the possible effects of diet on our ability to obtain quality sleep.

Of course, it could be the act of getting food, rather than what is in the food, that makes some food seem to relieve RLS. Many RLSers say they get relief from eating a banana. Bananas have potassium, and potassium relieves muscle cramps, but RLS symptoms usually do not involve muscle cramps. It might be that bananas are helpful because of their tryptophan content and their sleep-promoting ability, rather than because of their potassium, or bananas might be helpful because you have to get up, walk to the kitchen to get them, and then walk back to bed.

Some RLSers can drink coffee to relieve RLS symptoms, while others have to avoid caffeine entirely. Caffeine has also been thought to be the trigger for pain associated with RLS. Everyone is different, but there are enough reports on the negative effects of caffeine to warrant taking a good look at restricting it.

Even if caffeine does not trigger your RLS, keep in mind its effect on your ability to quickly get to sleep. The longer I lie awake in bed, the more chance I have of an RLS attack.

For this reason, I try to avoid caffeine after about 2:00 P.M. If I have it after that, it is only because I need to stay awake to drive or take part in an evening activity. Sleepiness will trigger my RLS, so if I have to stay awake for an evening activity, caffeine will ward off my sleepiness and keep the RLS at bay. The trouble with this is that once I've had a late dose of caffeine, it's a real trick to get to sleep that night.

Chocolate is an RLS trigger for many people. It could be a result of the caffeine or it could be from the tyramine in the chocolate. If you are one whose RLS is triggered by chocolate, you might want to look at the list of other foods high in caffeine or tyramine. Perhaps some of those foods are also RLS triggers for you.

Alcohol intake can affect sleep patterns and your ability to get to sleep. Some people claim a *little something* to drink will help them get to sleep. The trouble is that even though alcohol can make you sleepy, it can also cause restless sleep. Is it worth using it as a *going to sleep* trick, if it keeps you restless and causes multiple wake ups? If you must use alcohol, try to avoid red wine, which is often associated with RLS symptoms.

Quinine, in pills or as found in tonic water, has long been recommended for leg cramps associated with RLS symptoms. Some RLSers have sworn their prescription dose of quinine has helped reduce RLS symptoms. The response I see most often from RLS specialists and RLS literature is that quinine probably relieves a related muscular problem that might have been triggering RLS symptoms.

Since certain foods may help one person but be bad for another, there is no way to give you a list of what to eat and what to avoid. The point of this section is to encourage you to analyze how food affects your RLS symptoms. When you see patterns or results from certain foods, make your adjustments accordingly.

Be aware of your thoughts about getting to sleep

What are you thinking as you approach the bedtime hours?

You might be thinking, "I sure hope I don't have RLS symptoms tonight."

If the symptoms appear, are you disappointed, frustrated, or in a panic over getting to sleep?

Many RLSers have thoughts of dread and doom, such as, "I am afraid to go to bed, because I just know RLS will show up and keep me walking the floor all night."

These negative and victimizing thought patterns make things worse. We must expect RLS to be there when we get into bed and when we wake up during the night.

Though we should expect symptoms to appear, we need not fear them. Instead, we can be ready with a well-planned BOTA. Resist the tendency to allow your RLS symptoms to throw you into a panic. When RLS symptoms begin, be ready with your Plan of Attack and Relief Plans. Focus on your music, concentration techniques, or whatever tricks help you get to sleep. Maintain total confidence in your ability to get to sleep.

Try to avoid stressful thoughts before going to bed. Many sleep experts recommend taking the television out of the bedroom, avoiding the evening news, and steering clear of mind-bending thriller movies. Personally, I need to avoid movies or television shows that are choppy comedies or silly shows with someone getting deeper and deeper into trouble. A good mind-engaging show will actually relax my legs. Again, because we are all different, I offer these ideas to stimulate your thoughts rather than to suggest there is any best advice for everyone.

Develop your wind-down routine

Timing is critical to good sleep habits. Realize that if you plan to hit the pillow at 10:00 P.M., your wind-down routine might have to start at 9:00 P.M. Do the same routine every night. If you take evening medicines to avoid RLS symptoms or to induce sleep, consider what time they have to be in your system in order for them to be effective when needed. Also plan one last bathroom run to account for what you drank when you took your pills.

Your nightly routine might include household tasks, such as turning off house lights, locking doors, or checking your *to-do* list for the next day. Next, you might tend to personal hygiene in an effort to prepare your body for bed. Make sure your sinuses are clear so you can breathe easily during the night. Apply lotions so you are not bothered by itching from dry skin. Do what it takes to insure comfort and relaxation when you get into bed.

While tending to personal hygiene, be especially aware of your thinking. Concentrate on positive thoughts, such as, "I can't wait for my head to hit the pillow and my eyes to close. I am looking forward to a full night of sleep." Repeating positive thoughts during your wind-down routine will help prepare your mind and body for sleep.

Routinely prepare your room, setting up aroma therapy, checking room temperature, or turning on a fan or heater. Have a pad of paper available so you can make a list of things to think about in the morning. Leave your worries on the nightstand. They will be there for you in the morning. Avoid stressful or deep conversations as you head to bed. Make it a habit to get into bed, start your Plan of Attack, and go straight to sleep.

Although some sleep literature and surveys suggest it is not uncommon to take fifteen to twenty minutes to get to sleep, I believe RLSers should shoot for five minutes or less. At first, this won't happen, but eventually, with a well-prac-ticed Plan of Attack, it is very possible. The longer we are awake in bed, the greater chance we have of experiencing escalating RLS symptoms. The sooner we get to sleep, the better.

Use sleep-inducing words and images

As you think about going to bed, be aware of the individual words you use in your thoughts.

I set the stage for going straight to sleep, and staying asleep, when I tell myself, "I want to go out like a light and sleep soundly, until morning."

When I get into bed, I use specific words to ask myself, "Am I ready to *fall* asleep *now* and stay in a *deep* sleep until morning?"

The words *fall, now,* and *deep* suggest I will immediately tumble into a solid state of sleep.

Words can give us visual images that suggest thoughts or actions. With self-hypnosis, a person might be taught to picture an elevator going down one floor at a time and coming out way below, perhaps at a beach. At that bottom level, the person will be in a deep state of relaxation. The visual of going down relates strongly to *falling* asleep. If you use music to help you get to sleep, you might think of each song as taking you down another level. With this analogy, words like *fall* and *deep* become more meaningful. You can imagine yourself falling into bed and getting lost in your music, until you fall to the lowest level, where you will be in a deep sleep. You may still be aware of your thinking during the first few songs, but with each song, you will go lower and lower, or deeper and deeper, until you are deeply asleep.

When you are trying to overcome signals from the *RLS bully,* it is important to stay as focused as possible. Tell yourself you want to concentrate on every word and every instrumental sound until the very last sound of the last song. The more you stay focused on your music, the faster you will go to sleep.

Do not tell yourself, "I want to be asleep by the end of the first song." Instead, say, "I am going to focus and concentrate on every sound."

If your mind wanders, restart the song. Keep telling yourself to focus on every sound. Eventually, your subconscious will take over, causing you to fall asleep before the first song is finished.

The process is similar to reverse psychology. The more you tell yourself to remain consciously focused, the more your subconscious will take over and allow you to fall asleep. You will be shocked when you awake and can't remember hearing the last half of the album, even though your headphones are still on or your ear is still pressed to the pillow speaker.

Middle-of-the-night wake ups

Many RLSers report they can *get* to sleep, but they can't *stay* asleep. They also report they never feel refreshed after sleeping. If you are tired, even though you think you slept through the night, it could be a sign you are also dealing with PLMD, sleep apnea, or other sleep disorders that prevent quality sleep. A sleep study might give more information on the cause of your poor quality of sleep and periodic awakenings.

Some RLSers experience awakenings that seem to occur at the same time each night. If this is your problem, you can discuss it with your doctor or do some analytical experimentation. One idea is to view the wake-up cycle as a bad habit. Your body can get into a rhythmic and habitual behavior pattern that sets your body's time clock to keep waking you up. The task, then, is to discourage that habit and reset your body clock.

I have had several times when my body went into a cycle of waking every night at the same time. During one of these periods, I woke every night at exactly 2:20 A.M. I began wondering if a truck went by each night at exactly that time. I would wake up suddenly, look at the clock, and there it was, exactly 2:20 A.M. The one trick I found to break the 2:20 A.M. habit was to purposely stay up late for one night. When I broke my normal bedtime routine, I slept until a later hour and broke the cycle.

My rebellious way of looking at middle-of-the-night wake ups is to say it doesn't matter how many times you wake up. What matters is how fast you can get back to sleep. If you wake up during the night, quickly apply your Plan of Attack and get right back to sleep. If RLS symptoms begin, you may have to get out of bed to relieve them, but be quick about it and get right back to the task of getting to sleep. If your Plan of Attack fails, quickly employ a Relief Plan and stop the RLS symptoms. Then go right back to bed and use your best Plan of Attack. Have faith that whatever Plan of Attack you used at 10:00 P.M. will be just as reliable at 2:00 A.M. Insist on sleep. See yourself as a sleeper, not a nightwalker.

Some sleep specialists will treat middle-of-the-night awakenings with advice to avoid daytime naps. The idea is to be extremely tired when you go to bed at night. The problem is that extreme tiredness can aggravate RLS symptoms and prevent sleep. Other specialists will tell a person to sleep whenever possible. There are many theories, many of which are probably right for one person and wrong for someone else. Analyze yourself and your habits, and experiment safely.

Common middle-of-the-night mistakes

There are two mistakes we tend to make when developing middle-of-the-night Relief Plans. The first is to develop Relief Plan activities that are more enjoyable than going back to bed. The activities that help us calm RLS symptoms should not be ones that make us eager to be awake. If it has to be something we enjoy, like playing Solitaire, we need to be sure to go back to bed as soon as the RLS symptoms subside. I made this mistake many times, staying awake and losing precious sleep, just because I loved the quiet of the night and the peaceful feeling in my legs more than my restless moments in bed.

The second mistake RLSers have been known to make is to reserve routine chores to be completed during middle-of-the-night wake ups. One RLSer told me she would empty her dishwasher during her first wake-up period. The next time she awoke, she would fold the laundry. The next time, she would pay her bills.

I finally asked, "What if you didn't get up during the night?"

She looked at me and said, "That would be awful. I would never get my chores done."

Suddenly, she realized she had trained herself to be alert and ready for work during the night, rather than to be ready for sleep. From then on, she planned Relief Plans with unimportant activities (e.g., hot baths, playing Solitaire, stretching exercises).

Try some unpleasant Relief Plans

If your Relief Plans are more enticing than staying in bed and making your Plan of Attack work, you may have to develop some unpleasant Relief Plan activities.

You might tell yourself, "If I have to get out of bed a third time, I will do 100 heel lift stretches."

If that doesn't work, you might say Relief Plan #4 will be the unpleasant task of cleaning the toilet. Do whatever it takes to make sure you do not prefer Relief Plan activities to staying in bed and making your Plan of Attack work.

If you can't think of unpleasant activities for your Relief Plan, try creating a list of too many activities to enjoy. If the thought of doing all the activities is exhausting, you will eventually prefer to stay in bed and work harder at making your Plan of Attack work. Make a list of what you will do each time you get out of bed, and when you get out of bed, be committed to doing everything on the list. For example:

1. Go to the bathroom.
2. Do fifty heel lifts.
3. Make a cup of tea.
4. Do fifty heel lifts.
5. Drink the cup of tea.
6. Write one letter you have been putting off.
7. Do fifty heel lifts.
8. Go to the bathroom again.
9. Go back to bed and use your Plan of Attack.

After doing these activities every time you get out of bed, you will be tempted to skip parts or return to pleasant activities, like playing games on the computer. Force yourself to stick to your unpleasant Relief Plan activities. The goal is to get immediate RLS relief and encourage a desire to go to bed, apply your Plan of Attack, and get right to sleep.

You and your sleep partner

Numerous problems can arise when an RLSer shares a sleeping space. Some of the problems can be addressed by the RLSer, while others are better addressed by the partner. An upcoming chapter will give suggestions to help the partner deal with a loved one who has RLS. The following tips are meant to help the RLSer deal with issues involving a sleep partner.

1. **Communicate.** Do not expect your partner to know what hampers your ability to get to sleep. Explain a need for wiggle room or a tendency to have worse RLS if your

partner touches you as you fall asleep. If you pull away or sigh in frustration, you do not want your partner to take it personally. Tell your partner what helps and what makes things worse, so you can develop bedtime behaviors that help, rather than irritate.

2. **Avoid certain bedtime conversations.** Your partner may find bedtime conversations relaxing, but you might find they trigger RLS attacks. Analyze what types of conversations need to be avoided. You might want to avoid discussing plans for the next day, mentioning finances, or sharing fears and concerns.

3. **Try using two beds.** Many RLSers find it is better to have their own bed. Some couples use twin beds pushed together. If you want to maintain the look of a single bed, you can use a king-size bedspread over the twin beds. Many RLSers also have Periodic Limb Movement Disorder, causing them to thrash around during their sleep. If you are in this situation, you might have to pull the twin beds slightly apart so your movements don't shake your partner's bed.

4. **Who goes first?** Experiment with whether it is best for you to get to sleep before your partner. If my husband gets to sleep before me, my RLS symptoms can be aggravated by my attempts to be still and not wake him. Sometimes it's better for me to get to bed first and begin dozing before he gets to bed.

5. **Try the *partner pin*.** Most RLSers are vehemently opposed to anything preventing their free movement in bed. There are some of us, however, who occasionally like it if our partner cuddles closely and throws a leg over ours, pinning us down. If the timing is just right, it can keep us settled and help us get to sleep. Other times, that same trick is the worst thing in the world. If you have good communication with your partner, it will be

understandable when you declare it a bad night for the *partner pin*.

6. **Support your partner.** Try to understand the frustrations RLS issues create for your partner. Share the upcoming chapter, designed to help those who support RLSers. The more our partners understand about RLS and the more they feel competent in their ability to support us, the easier RLS survival will be for everyone.

    These days, when I "ootch and scrootch" in bed, my husband no longer huffs and puffs with irritated frustration. He gently moves away and waits for me to tell him whether it's safe to move back. Sometimes I tell him to try again, but sometimes we both know it's best to give a hug, move apart, and go to sleep on our own. That kind of mutual understanding goes a long way toward helping both of us get a good night's sleep.

7. **Get comfortable.** Make sure you and your sleep partner have plenty of room and are comfortable. The tendency of most RLSers is to avoid being touched, cramped, or boxed in. In an effort to have our own space, we do something that can make things worse: we get as close to our edge of the bed as possible. How can we get to sleep when we are pinning ourselves tightly to the edge of the bed and laying there in a panic over whether our space will be crowded? The following section gives a solution to this problem.

The *snuggle trick*

Instead of cowering at the edge of your bed, try the *snuggle trick*. Be the first one into bed, and immediately scoot over to your partner's side of the bed. Allow just enough room for your partner to get into bed. When your partner gets into bed, snuggle for as long as you can. Make sure your legs stay on top so you are free to move when you are ready to stop snuggling.

I can usually snuggle for five to ten minutes, but sometimes it's only a minute or two before the first RLS urge strikes and I know it is time to end the snuggle. Most of the time, the snuggle ends just when our breathing changes and we begin drifting off to sleep. At that point, we hug, kiss, and roll away from each other. He rolls over to his edge of the bed, which is not far for him to go. I roll over and claim all the rest of the bed for myself. That leaves me about two-thirds of the bed to kick around in without bothering my partner. As you can see, there is a method to my madness.

The Author's BOTA
for Getting to Sleep

THE BAG OF Tricks Approach (BOTA) is a relatively simple concept to understand, but can be a challenge to put into action. First, you need to become familiar with the steps of the BOTA: Gather Your Tricks, Pack Your Bags, Plan of Attack, and Relief Plans. Then you must figure out how the steps fit together and how you can apply them as a strategy that works for you night after night.

I am often asked what supplements I use, what aggravators I've identified, or what tricks I use to get to sleep. I hesitate to give specifics of my situation, because I want people to figure out what works for them, rather than copying what works for me. Nevertheless, in light of the fact the BOTA can be tricky to apply and because *getting to sleep* is one of the most important activities to master, I have decided to offer an example of my own BOTA for getting to sleep.

The following example will show you how all the steps of the BOTA fit together and how Step 3: Plan of Attack and Step 4: Relief Plans can be repeated until sleep is achieved. Remember, it is just an example of what I have used. The props and strategies I use now are different than ones I used when I was first developing my BOTA. The example below is a combination of things I have used over the years. I am not suggesting you use my tricks or follow my Plan of Attack and Relief Plans. Pay attention to how I apply the steps, but imagine your own favorite tricks being used.

BOTA Step 1: Gather Your Tricks
(for all RLS situations)

In the *Gather Your Tricks* section of my RLS Rebel Program notebook, I list tricks for many at-rest activities. The following lists of tricks are just a sampling.

No-prop tricks: a good wind-down routine, positive thoughts, stretching, concentration (usually picturing myself doing a clog dancing routine), *bully noise, zero tolerance,* walking, dancing, brushing, imaginary *RLS rubbing cream,* controlled breathing, sex, the *snuggle trick,* simulated walking while seated, using my foot to draw letters of the alphabet in the air.

Prop tricks: Tension Tamer tea, massage with lavender cream, headphones with favorite CD, pillow speaker, aroma therapy, computer games, hot tub, supplements, vibrator/massager, hypnosis CD, suckers, popcorn, therapy bands, knitting, piano playing.

Tricks I might try in the future: prescription medicines, a bar of soap under the sheet, air wraps that squeeze my legs (like the ones hospitals use to prevent blood clots).

BOTA Step 2: Pack Your Bags
(for getting to sleep)

The contents of my BOT for getting to sleep can vary. I might choose one set of tricks for getting to sleep when I am home, but another set of tricks for getting to sleep while on a trip (e.g., in a hotel, at someone's house, in a recreational vehicle). The following is an example of a BOT I might use at home. The no-prop list helps me remember options that do not have visual representations. The prop list reminds me what items I need to have for my Plan of Attack and Relief Plans.

No-Prop Tricks (for getting to sleep): wind-down routine, *snuggle trick,* positive thoughts, wiggling, deep breaths, concentration, dancing.

Prop Tricks (for getting to sleep): computer Solitaire, herbal tea, cold drink, aroma spray, supplements, headphones, CD player and favorite CD, hot tub, lotion.

BOTA Step 3: Plan of Attack
(for getting to sleep)

Remember, there are two parts to the Plan of Attack: prepare and attack. First, I take steps to ensure I will start the activity with the least chance of being disturbed by RLS symptoms. Then I apply tricks that help me get through the activity, despite any RLS symptoms that might appear.

PREPARE: My preparation for going to sleep begins early in the evening. Ideally, I keep to a routine bedtime, around 10:00 P.M. If my husband reads this, he will laugh out loud. If it were not for his discipline of sticking to a bedtime, I probably wouldn't know what *routine bedtime* meant. Even when I have a bedtime in mind, I often forget to start early so I can keep to that schedule. If I fail to start early, skipping my wind-down routine and jumping right into bed, there is a good chance I will not be able to relax and get to sleep.

In my best wind-down routine, I begin by cleaning up the kitchen and checking my calendar so I am prepared for the next day's activities. I might find a chore I can finish quickly so I feel accomplished and settled. Then I might make a cup of herbal relaxation tea and drink it slowly, while I play my favorite computer game, Spider Solitaire. I try to play at a level where I can easily win. It is important that I win, so I go to bed feeling powerful, not frustrated and helpless.

Then I shut down the computer and mosey toward the bedroom. I might take a cold drink to my bedside, turn on some music, or spray something that smells good on my pillow. Next, my bathroom routine might include physical hygiene routines, along with taking my nighttime supplements. If I took routine prescription medications for RLS, I might take them at this point in my routine. If the medicines need more than ten to twenty minutes to go to work, I would need to take them before starting the computer game.

During all of this wind-down routine, I try to replace the worries of the day with thoughts of my blessings. I think back to all I accomplished that day and recount all the nice things that happened. The idea is to feel as satisfied and as finished with the day as possible. I consciously think positive thoughts about going to bed. As I described in the last chapter, my choice of words is very important.

Some helpful thoughts might be: "I am looking forward getting into my comfortable bed. I can't wait to fall into a deep sleep. Tonight, I will go to sleep quickly and sleep soundly until morning."

ATTACK: I try to get to sleep before RLS symptoms have a chance to start. Even if no RLS symptoms are present, I always follow the five steps of my attack phase: 1) Wiggle, 2) Take two deep breaths, 3) Ask the question, 4) Start *bully noise*, and 5) Use *zero tolerance*.

1. **Wiggle.** Sometimes my *attack* begins with the *snuggle trick*. Other times, I start with the end of the trick where I move back to my part of the bed, purposefully wiggle, and explore my space. It is intentional squirming, even though I am not experiencing an urge to move. I figure, I might as well check out my space and make sure there is plenty of room, in case I need to squirm. I make sure the covers are loose and my husband's legs and arms are not invading my space.

2. **Take two deep breaths.** I take two fast, deep, cleansing breaths. If I forget this step, I will usually discover I am tense and subconsciously preventing sleep. Without the deep breaths, it is as if I am still holding on to the day and afraid to let it go. After breathing deeply, I feel surrendered, glued to the mattress, and ready to be still.

The two breaths I use are not slow, relaxing breaths. If I were to slowly breathe in and out, I would surely have an RLS attack. These are fast and furious breaths that would make someone wonder about me if they heard them. Be sure to tell your sleep partner that the noisy breaths are part of your plan and a sign you are within minutes of being sound asleep.

3. **Ask the question.** This might seem silly, but I find it helpful to ask myself, "Am I ready to go to sleep, now?"

   There is a natural desire to hold onto my thoughts, lest I forget something important. If I am not willing to relax and make a conscious decision to put my worries aside until morning, I can't possibly be ready to go to sleep.

   When I first worked at putting my thoughts aside, I tried a principle used with worry dolls. These are tiny figures you can keep by your bedside. The idea is to tell the dolls all your worries, so they can hold them for you until morning. Similarly, there is a lovely saying: "Before you go to sleep at night, give all your worries to God. He will be up all night, anyhow."

   If I have made several unsuccessful attempts to get to sleep and have to intersperse several Relief Plans, I sometimes ask myself two questions.

   The first is the usual, "Am I ready to go to sleep now?"

   Because I can easily get in the habit of quickly answering that question without carefully thinking about my readiness, I ask the second question, "Is that my final answer?"

   If the answer is no, I get out of bed, take care of the thoughts I can't seem to relinquish, and then return to bed and start my Plan of Attack again.

4. **Start *bully noise*.** After years of practice, I have confidence that *bully noise* will work for me. If I allow my

mind to follow random thoughts, I am sure to have RLS attacks, so I clutter my thoughts with music or concentration. My best trick is to turn on my CD player and listen to my *Meatloaf* CD. If I don't have the CD player, I use the no-prop trick of concentrating on one of my clogging routines. If my mind wanders, I start back at the beginning, as many times as necessary, forcing myself to concentrate. Two earlier chapters have detailed information on using concentration and music.

5. **Use *zero tolerance*.** During a bad RLS attack, *bully noise* may not be enough to overpower the irresistible urges to move. If my RLS symptoms keep getting worse, I quickly apply the best trick of all, *zero tolerance*. I get out of bed and quickly start my first Relief Plan.

BOTA Step 4: Relief Plans
(for stopping symptoms)

I have several Relief Plans that become increasingly more involved and more reliable. The first time my Plan of Attack fails, I use the shortest and easiest Relief Plan. It is designed as a distraction to allow me to get right back to bed and try my Plan of Attack again. Later, the more involved Relief Plans focus on calming the RLS symptoms and waiting for my body to relax and be ready for sleep.

First Relief Plan: Get up, go to the bathroom, get a drink of water, and go back to bed. Try the Plan of Attack again.

Second Relief Plan: Get up, walk to the other side of the house, stretch a little, dance a few clogging steps, check my *to-do* list, and go back to bed. Try the Plan of Attack again.

Third Relief Plan: Get up, make some Tension Tamer herbal tea (two bags, in sixteen ounces of water, allowing the bags to steep until the last medicinal sip), play twenty minutes of computer games, massage my legs with lavender cream, and go back to bed. Try the Plan of Attack again.

Fourth Relief Plan: Get up, soak in the hot tub (staying there until I am relaxed and starting to doze), and go back to bed. Try the Plan of Attack again.

Fifth and Final Relief Plan: Get up, pay bills until 4:00 A.M., and go back to bed. Try the Plan of Attack again.

My fifth Relief Plan is usually my final plan, because after 4:00 A.M. I am almost always able to get to sleep. Many RLSers, even on a really bad night, can finally get to sleep after 4:00 A.M. The tendency is to give up and figure you will not get any sleep, but it is important to try your Plan of Attack one more time. Even if you get only an hour of sleep before the alarm goes off, it will be worth it.

Many people look at this plan and think it has no benefit if it means I might be awake all night doing Relief Plans, but in fact, there are many benefits. First, I become more skillful with each repetition of my Plan of Attack. Second, I build confidence in my ability to stop RLS attacks with one of my reliable Relief Plans. And third, I avoid panic, aimless floor walking, and feelings of being a helpless victim. Usually, I am asleep after the first or second Relief Plan. Regardless of how many Relief Plans I need, it is important to take control and stick to my plan.

When I am confident my Relief Plans work, I am finally able to relax and really put my efforts into my Plan of Attack. Sometimes, even when the Plan of Attack fails, I remind myself I can always get out of bed and start another Relief Plan or I can make one more careful attempt to make the Plan of Attack work. Many times, that second Plan of Attack does the job.

I began this program having to use all my Relief Plans and waiting until 4:00 A.M. on many nights. Eventually, I was able to get to sleep 90 percent of the time with one good Plan of Attack and no Relief Plans. That's the goal, but it takes time, patience, discipline, and lots of repetition before you build the skills and confidence to have that kind of success. It all pays off in time, and it is well worth the effort.

Special Situations

WHEN I INITIALLY told my friends and family about RLS, I was asked, "Is that why you always insist on driving? Is that why you go to bed so late? Is that why you always ask for aisle seats?"

Answering all the questions with yes, I was amazed at how many subconscious adjustments I was accustomed to making in order to accommodate the obnoxious urges to wiggle. Today, my adjustments for RLS are conscious and carefully planned.

RLSers can be skillful at accommodating their RLS symptoms during normal daily activities, but not know what to do when special situations arise. Many people have to plan ahead for handicap accessibility, making sure they will be comfortable and able to function in an upcoming situation. Likewise, RLSers need to think ahead to what will make special RLS-provoking situations more bearable. The following are special situations that call for a little different information, preparation, and response than normal.

Hospitalizations

When planning hospital stays, many RLSers find it helpful to discuss RLS issues with their doctors, and to have notes about RLS added to their charts. The information may include lists of drugs to avoid and recommended substitute drugs. A short description of RLS symptoms and related patient behavior might also be noted. Addressing these topics before a hospital stay can facilitate communication and pre-vent situations which aggravate RLS symptoms.

An RLS Medical Alert Card is a handy way to bring RLS information to the attention of doctors, nurses, and other hospital personnel. The cards are wallet-sized explana-tions of what medicines to avoid and what medicines are relatively safe for RLSers. The cards also give a brief descrip-tion of RLS and RLSers' behaviors. The following websites have information on obtaining the cards. Each source has a slightly different card, but they all cover the same general information.

http://www.legsmove.org/med-card.htm
(San Antonio Support Group)

http://www.rlshelp.org
(Southern California Support Group)

http://www.rls.org
(The Restless Legs Syndrome Foundation)

If you take medications for RLS, you will need to ask whether they can be continued during your hospitaliza-tion. Discuss your usual regimen with your doctor and ask to have it noted in your hospital charts. Many RLSers have found it helpful to have their own copy of orders for medi-cations or supplements they want to take or avoid while in the hospital.

While your doctor is adding RLS-related information to your hospital charts, ask him to add a short description of RLS behavior and a warning to avoid patient confinement. Your frantic efforts to kick off tight covers or wiggle should not be viewed as hysteria or defiance. If you request your headphones and music, it should be seen as a necessary RLS treatment rather than an optional activity. When I awoke from surgery, I immediately asked to have my headphones and music. The ICU nurse told me I would have to wait until

I was moved to my hospital room. After I told her to check the RLS notes in my chart, she made sure I had my music available immediately.

For a few days after surgery, while still using pain killers, most RLSers find they are RLS-free. However, when the pain medicines are discontinued, the RLS symptoms often seem to come back with a vengeance. Before assuming your RLS is worse than ever, take an inventory of your situation and try getting back to what you were doing for RLS prior to your hospital stay. Reinstate supplement regimens, exercise programs, and bedtime routines that may have been interrupted during your hospital stay. Revisit the steps of the Reduction Plan and see if there are any new variables resulting from your hospitalization, illness, or medications. Use your best Plan of Attacks, repeating the detailed steps you used when you first started controlling your RLS. It may take time to get back to your good habits.

Disasters and accidents

As a child, before I knew there was a name for *my leg thing*, I learned about people hiding from the Nazis. I couldn't help but wonder what people would do if their legs bothered them and they had to stretch while in hiding. What would they do in a tiny cramped space if their lives depended upon their staying still and being totally quiet?

Another frightening scenario was the thought of breaking a leg and having to spend six weeks in a full leg cast. How would a person wiggle and stretch inside a cast? It seemed as though it would be enough to drive an RLSer insane. A rehabilitation/recovery situation might be good reason to rely heavily on one form or another of a prescription medication. Music, self-hypnosis, and other distraction tricks would also be good responses to RLS attacks if movement were not an option.

There are many other situations that could cause sudden immobility. What if you were trapped under wreckage from an accident, hurricane, or terrorist attack? What if you couldn't get up and walk, reach your legs to massage them, or take your medication? There is a good chance adrenaline, fear, pain, and distraction would prevent or overpower RLS symptoms. Otherwise, the no-prop tricks of concentration and *bully noise* might be your best bet.

Kidney disease and dialysis

End-stage kidney disease is known to trigger severe and unmanageable secondary RLS. Even when RLSers have had control over their primary RLS symptoms, they can suddenly find themselves unable to manage symptoms aggravated by kidney disease and lengthy dialysis treatments. People who have never had RLS symptoms can suddenly experience a case of secondary RLS, caused by their kidney disease. With no previous knowledge of RLS and no experience facing symptoms, they are often caught totally off guard and unprepared to respond to symptoms.

Years ago, I corresponded with a doctor who had RLS and was well known for his tireless support of RLSers. When his kidney disease progressed and dialysis treatments were needed, his RLS symptoms became more severe than anything he had ever experienced. To aggravate matters, the long drive to his treatment center triggered RLS attacks that left him frustrated and anxious. By the time he sat down for several hours of dialysis, none of his usual tricks were effective against his raging RLS symptoms.

In an effort to help, I suggested he ease his symptoms by exercising before dialysis, sucking on suckers, listening to music, concentrating, doing self-massage (or getting someone to give him a massage), using warm or cold compresses, and avoiding caffeine. He tried all the suggestions and used several medications, but experienced no relief. His panic, frustration, and sense of helplessness appeared to be overpowering his confidence and ability to control his RLS. To his credit, the disease may have caused more symptoms than any Bag of Tricks (BOT) could handle.

When I imagine dealing with RLS and dialysis, I become even more determined to perfect tricks like self-hypnosis and *bully noise*. I hope new RLS treatments will be discovered, making dialysis more bearable for RLSers. If you are facing dialysis, be sure to educate your doctor about RLS and to retrieve all the latest ideas from the RLS Foundation and other RLS specialists on ways to manage RLS while facing end-stage kidney disease and dialysis.

Chemotherapy

Chemotherapy treatments do not bring the forced immobility seen with dialysis. Typically, a person's medicine bags are hung from a portable IV pole and the person must be attached to the bags' tubing until all the chemicals have been infused. Fortunately, chemotherapy patients are able to move around, as long as they drag the IV pole with them. Of course, a patient's health might not allow for walking, but the person might have the option to move and stretch while remaining seated.

Though mobility might not be an issue with chemotherapy, pre-meds and chemotherapy drugs can create safety concerns and aggravate RLS symptoms. Anti-nausea medicines can cause drowsiness, effect balance, and produce fluctuations in blood pressure, making walking a hazardous endeavor. Some commonly administered pre-meds (e.g., Benadryl, Phenergan, Compazine) are known to trigger RLS symptoms. Chemotherapy patients can avoid RLS attacks if their doctors substitute medicines that are less likely to trigger RLS attacks.

Pregnancy

Women with primary RLS often experience more severe symptoms during pregnancy. It is also common for pregnant women who have never experienced RLS symptoms to suddenly be bothered by them. In both cases, symptoms during pregnancy would be considered a secondary case of RLS. There is actually quite a bit of literature on RLS during pregnancy, including recommendations to manage ferritin and folic acid levels. Be sure to get the latest information on dealing with RLS during pregnancy.

Secondary RLS symptoms experienced during pregnancy usually subside after delivery. However, many women continue to be plagued by their primary RLS symptoms while nursing their babies or while rocking their babies to sleep. If you are nursing a baby and bothered by RLS symptoms, experiment with various positions to nurse or rock your baby so you are free to wiggle or move away without disturbing the baby. You might find it easiest to nurse on your side, leaving yourself free to wiggle or move away when your baby falls asleep.

If prescription medications have been one of your main RLS tricks, you will want to discuss the safety of using those medications while pregnant or nursing. Music, audio books, or suckers may help by creating mental distractions while rocking a baby to sleep. As you analyze the situation, think of all the tricks in your BOT and think creatively about how you might use them while caring for your baby.

When an RLSer is bedridden

There are many reasons an RLSer might be bedridden and faced with severe RLS symptoms that are difficult to relieve. If an illness creates a situation where you must have a caregiver heavily involved in your care, be sure to educate that person about RLS behavior and the importance of using *zero tolerance* and *bully noise*. Your caregiver can learn to spot restlessness movements and quickly distract you or help you wiggle safely (see the upcoming chapter "To Those Who Support Us").

Many RLSers report that sleep medicines make them drowsy but do not always stop raging RLS attacks and the need to walk. A dangerous situation exists when medications, extended bed rest, or illness interferes with a person's balance and stability. If you must walk under these conditions, be sure you have assistance.

If walking is not an option, a special BOT will be needed. You might be able to use music as a concentration trick. Massage can be comforting and effective in reducing RLS symptoms. Warm towel wraps or tub soaks can be soothing and distracting. Distraction can be a very useful trick, created by stimulating conversation, heated discussions, word puzzles, computerized games, or handicrafts (e.g., knitting, needlepoint, crocheting, drawing).

Even if you are bedridden, you can still apply the RLS Rebel Program. Use the Reduction Plan to analyze new variables that might be unique to being bedridden. Attempt to reduce the *RLS beast* to an *RLS bully*. Develop a Bag of Tricks Approach (BOTA) for preventing and responding to RLS symptoms that attack while you are in bed. If you are anticipating becoming bedridden (perhaps due to an upcoming surgery), plan ahead and be ready with a special BOTA.

Work situations

I was surprised one day, after speaking to an RLS support group, when a man told me he did not see how any of my ideas could be applied to the RLS symptoms that plagued him at his job. His work required him to sit at a computer for eight hours a day. He thought everything I had talked about had to do with sleeping, watching television, or at-home activities.

Under the American Disabilities Act (ADA), RLSers are entitled to receive special consideration for some issues relating to RLS. With some relatively simple adjustments, the principles of the Reduction Plan and BOTA can be applied, limiting aggravating variables and providing a plan for preventing and responding to RLS symptoms. The following is a list of suggestions that can help you deal with RLS in the workplace and help your workplace remain compliant with the ADA.

1. Adjust or exchange your chair, trying various heights and densities of seats. Experiment with lumbar supports and consider the differences in stationary chairs and ones that rock or swivel.

2. Change your work schedule. Even if RLS symptoms are not a problem at work, sleepless nights may cause exhaustion, which prevents your ability to accomplish your job or carry out tasks safely. If your best sleep is from 4:00 a.m. to 9:00 a.m., you may do better going to work in the late morning. If your RLS is worse in the afternoon, you may do better on a morning shift. If you sit for part of the day and move around freely for the rest of the time, try scheduling seated activities for the mornings, when you are less likely to have RLS attacks.

3. Take regular breaks, even if they are every fifteen minutes and just long enough to stand, touch your toes, or walk to the other side of the room and back. If possible, use *zero tolerance*, standing up and stopping the RLS attacks the minute they start.

4. Use a two-chambered air pillow or stepping device under your desk to simulate walking while still doing your job, or do the same motion without the pillow (i.e., putting both feet on the floor and pressing them alternately

to the ground), so the thigh muscles work as if you were walking.

5. Use headphones to listen to music or white noise.

6. Use a vibrating heated chair cushion.

7. Suck on suckers.

8. Use herbal teas to reduce tension. Be careful to not use ones that induce sleep.

9. Use a well-planned BOTA. Know what tricks you will use, and be ready to prevent and respond to RLS symptoms at your desk. If your Plan of Attack fails, have your first Relief Plan ready to go.

10. Educate your boss and co-workers, being sure they understand RLS is a recognized disability. Explain how you will do your best to control it without disturbing others. Stress your commitment to your responsibilities, even though your actions may look as if you are less than focused on the job. Discuss the importance of *zero tolerance* and the risks of putting off movement when RLS symptoms occur.

Theaters/movies/concerts

Two or three hours of sitting and watching a show can be a real test for an RLS rebel. Certain snacks can provide helpful distractions (e.g., popcorn, peanuts, raisins, candy). At a movie theater, I always get a bag of popcorn, even if I am not hungry. It's a great way to keep my mind off sitting still while I wait for the movie to grab my attention.

Consider the advantages of sitting near the back or side of the room, in case you have to resort to a Relief Plan and stand for a while. Try to reserve aisle seats or get there early enough to claim seats with easy escape routes. Always locate the exit doors and plan your best escape route, in case you need to go for a walk or do some serious stretching. Knowing you have a place you can find in the dark (i.e., where you can stand, stretch, or wiggle without bothering others) will help a great deal to prevent panic.

My favorite seats are in theaters with stadium-style seating. I love sitting in the first row of an upper level so I can put my feet on the metal dividing bars. Along with providing a great foot rest, the first row gives a sense of openness, rather than a feeling of being trapped in a crowded row.

If you can't get an aisle seat, try leaving a space between you and the people on either side. The extra room can prevent anxiety that might lead to RLS symptoms. I try to make the seat next to me look occupied, piling my coat and purse there, if possible. If someone asks to sit next to me when there are plenty of other seats available, I explain I have a disorder that prevents me from sitting still. Once they realize I may be too much of a distraction, they are usually happy to find another seat.

Several other adjustments can help you get through a movie or show, despite RLS symptoms. You may want to prepare for the event by wearing comfortable clothing, including shoes you can slip on and off. Try attending events in the early afternoon, when you are less likely to have uncontrollable RLS symptoms. Avoid overeating or consuming foods that may leave you uncomfortable during the show. If you are extremely tired, it might help to take a short nap before attending a movie or show. If you experience unruly RLS symptoms during a show, close your eyes and doze for a few minutes. You will miss part of the show, but the short nap may calm you and relieve RLS symptoms. Just be careful to not slide off the seat or snore too loudly.

Stroke and paralysis

Many RLSers have said their RLS symptoms were severe enough to make them want to cut off their legs. The follow-up comment is usually that they would have done it, if they weren't so sure they would have phantom RLS and then not be able to relieve their symptoms by walking. This dark humor is not far from the reality for RLSers who have suffered paralysis. A paralyzed person, such as a stroke survivor, is likely to have RLS symptoms and not have the benefit of being able to walk. Though we always consider walking to be a no-prop trick, when you think of it in this light, you might consider your legs to be essential props, thus making walking a prop trick.

If you are paralyzed and experiencing RLS symptoms, work closely with your healthcare provider to determine whether you are taking medications or receiving treatments that could be aggravating RLS symptoms. Also ask about prescription treatments that might alleviate symptoms. Remember to make use of tricks that do not require use of your paralyzed limbs (e.g., music, massage, concentration, mental distractions). If you have a caregiver, educate the person about your RLS symptoms and suggest helpful tricks to try (e.g., distracting you, giving you a massage, helping you move your limbs to relieve symptoms).

Exhaustion and personal safety

Sleep deprivation and side effects from medications can turn normal daily activities into special RLS situations. Exhaustion can lead to drowsiness, depression, and an inability to make good decisions about personal safety. Care should be taken when driving, operating machinery, or dealing with stressful situations. There are times when it is best to recognize the severity of your sleep deprivation and put an activity off until you are rested.

If you care for young children and you are not getting enough sleep, exhaustion can become a safety concern for you and the children. When my children were young, I was not aware that my restless sleep patterns were affecting my daily energy. I just knew I had a hard time staying awake and safely fulfilling my parenting duties.

Looking back, there were many days when I should have asked a neighbor or friend to watch the children while I caught up on my rest. That would have been safer than allowing my eyes to close and hoping to open them before the children could get into trouble. I had no idea how dangerous my lack of sleep could be to my children.

Sleep deprivation and frustration can have serious effects on a person's emotional state and desire to live. Many RLSers claim to have suicidal thoughts, brought on by their exhaustion and frustration with RLS symptoms. If you are one of these people, ask for help immediately.

Traveler's RLS

In many cases, people who already have their RLS under control during normal daily activities find themselves concerned about the special situation created by a long airline flight or several days of car travel. Long trips can be quite bearable if time is taken to carefully review the RLS Rebel Program's Reduction Plan and BOTA. The following chapter will further address the issue of traveling with RLS.

Traveler's RLS

THE FIRST TIME I heard the term *traveler's RLS* was at a 2004 meeting of the Restless Legs Syndrome Foundation. The special situation created by travel was recognized for its ability to aggravate RLS symptoms beyond an RLSer's normal daily experience. A person might have relatively mild RLS most of the time, but suddenly experience severe RLS symptoms when taking a long plane trip. A normal Bag of Tricks Approach (BOTA) might not be sufficient to prevent or respond to the unusually severe symptoms occurring during long trips. Therefore, RLSers should give special consideration to their BOTA before attempting to travel long distances.

The suggestions in this chapter were developed in response to RLSers who have contacted me over the years in a panic over the prospect of an upcoming trip. Though most of their concerns (and the concerns in the remainder of this chapter) were about airplane travel, our conversations resulted in suggestions that can easily be applied to other forms of travel. All the RLSers reported wonderful trips to their destinations after they carefully analyzed their travel Bag of Tricks, Plan of Attacks, and Relief Plans. Note that I said they had wonderful trips *to their destinations*. It is often the return trip that causes the most trouble.

Stowing your travel BOT

As you gather your prop tricks, think about where you will stow them during your trip. Make sure your props fit into a bag that can be stowed under the airplane seat in front of you. Remember, the area under a seat is smaller than the size restrictions for carryon luggage. If you already have a personal item to take onboard, consider putting your BOT in your larger carryon and removing it just before you board the airplane. Another idea is to put your personal item in a tote bag, along with your tricks, and count the whole bag as your personal item.

In most bulkhead rows and some exit rows, you may not be able to keep your BOT with you during take off and landing. As soon as you are in the air and the *Fasten Seat Belt* sign is turned off, you should be able to retrieve your bag from the overhead compartment. This might be good reason to avoid bulkhead rows and some exit rows. When in doubt, check with the airline about the rules on your flight.

I usually want my BOT stored under the seat in front of me. However, I often wonder if I'm creating a situation of: Which came first, the chicken or the egg? Do RLS symptoms start because I limit my leg room, or would I have RLS anyhow and be better off having my tricks close by? I figure it is best to have a full BOT within reach, always assuming RLS symptoms will appear.

Pack your travel BOT

As you are packing your BOT, take into account the weight, size, and potential usefulness of each prop. You do not want a bag that is too heavy to carry or too large to stow. You also do not want to be without a trick if you are left in a restrictive situation longer than expected. Would you have enough effective tricks if take-off were detained and you were confined to your seat while waiting for clearance? Consider the following items when packing your travel BOT.

1. **Thermal mug:** I usually pack a thermal mug with two herbal tea bags and sweetener already in it. Hot water is added later (see "Plan of Attack: The *preparation stage*" later in this chapter). The type of herbal tea depends on whether I want to promote sleep or just prevent tension. I always have extra tea bags and sweetener in my BOT, but I seldom need more than the first mug of tea.

2. **CDs, DVDs, tapes, MP3 players, and video cameras:** My travel BOT usually includes a portable CD player, earphones, and CDs with my favorite music. You might want to consider taking along (or renting at the airport) a DVD player and a good movie. Audio books can also be helpful in preventing RLS attacks. Be aware, however, that certain types of story lines can aggravate RLS. For me, slapstick themes or ones where the characters get deeper and deeper into trouble will drive my RLS crazy. A video camera can be used as a distraction if you use it to watch videos, such as ones you took while on the trip. Make sure to have fully charged batteries or extra non-rechargeable batteries for your audio/visual equipment. Earphones can be plugged into cameras and other equipment, making it possible to hear audio above the airplane noise.

3. **Reading, writing, and handwork:** Reading is an RLS aggravator for many, while other RLSers find a good book relaxing. Be aware of what types of reading material aggravate your RLS. The magazines on airplanes will usually trigger my RLS symptoms, whereas an intriguing novel might keep me well distracted and RLS free. Knitting, crossword puzzles, or a deck of cards can provide good distractions. Remember, some of these activities require props that might not be allowed past security checkpoints or during take-off and landing.

4. **Food and drink:** In addition to your personal item and normal carryon bag, you are allowed to take food to eat while on the airplane. Eating can be a wonderful way to prevent RLS symptoms, but consider how it might affect people around you. The aroma of pizza, Mexican food, or a hot pastrami sandwich can turn you into the most disliked person on the airplane. Prepare to fend off the glares and comments.

   I once opened a warm Mexican dinner and heard the person behind me groan, "It smells like someone's dirty socks!"

   The meal looked a little less appetizing with dirty socks in mind.

   Non-alcoholic drinks are also allowed as carryon items. I always try to have a bottle of water with me so I do not have to wait for the drink service. It took me awhile to learn to buy (or fill) the bottle of water near the gate so I did not have to lug the extra two or three pounds of water in my carryon bag. Be sure to use cups or bottles that can be closed securely.

5. **Snacks:** For RLS purposes, there is a difference between *food* and *snacks*. Consider using special snacks that last a long time and keep you busy (e.g., suckers, raisins, peanuts, popcorn). Something that requires you to open shells and manage the trash is even better (e.g., sunflower seeds, pistachio nuts). The bags of peanuts you get on some planes seem impossible to open, but if you take your time, they will provide a great distraction.

   Do not make the mistake one frustrated person did and yell, "Does anyone have a knife?"

6. **Comfort items:** Take along items that will help you feel comfortable. I usually have an inflatable neck pillow that helps when I decide to take a snooze. I still have not figured out how to keep my mouth from dropping open

or how to prevent drooling, but at least my head doesn't bounce around and my neck doesn't ache.

If you are taking a long car trip, I highly recommend trying a vibrating heated seat cushion. They feel good, relax you, and are even a good distraction, especially when the vibrations stop after a set time and then pop on to remind you to turn the power off. The sudden jolt is a great distraction. There are many portable cushions that can make car or airplane travel more comfortable and help ward off RLS symptoms. Be sure to check out the latest products.

7. **Stretch and exercise tools:** In an earlier chapter on prop tricks, I described a two-chambered air cushion that helps simulate walking while you are seated. There are also mini-stepping gadgets with two foot pads you press alternately. Some stepping units are small enough to put in a purse or pocket. Remember, some of the motions you get with these devices can be simulated without the device, making it a great no-prop trick.

   I usually pack an elastic therapy band in my travel BOT. When I get the urge to wiggle, the band helps me stretch my arms and legs without having to leave my seat. The band is lightweight and takes up very little space. For more information, see the earlier chapter "Prop Tricks: Non-Prescriptions."

8. **Medications and supplements:** If you will need supplements or RLS medications during your trip, be sure to keep them with you. You never know when delays might occur, luggage could be lost, or a sudden case of RLS may make you wish you had your medicines handy. I usually pack enough for a few extra days, in case of delays or changes in plans.

   Be cautious about what containers you use for your prescription medications and supplements. It's usually best to keep them in original labeled containers so there are no problems going through security checkpoints or customs. Despite that advice, I use plastic, resealable snack bags to organize my supplements for three weeks at a time. I never thought much about pulling them out and leaving bags on the bathroom counter in my hotel room until I saw a news report about drug trafficking in hotels. Many hotels in my area were training their cleaning staff to report guest rooms where they found piles of empty resealable snack bags. Now I hide mine. Can you imagine the scene if my vitamin C and calcium caused my arrest?

9. **No-prop tricks:** Remember to make note of your no-prop tricks when you are packing your BOT for travel. Massage, brushing (using imaginary rubbing cream), and concentration are all valuable tricks to have in your virtual travel BOT. They weigh nothing and you never have problems with them going through security checkpoints or being out of reach.

Plan of Attack: *Preparation stage*

Your Plan of Attack (for getting through the activity of sitting still on an airplane) should begin with a *preparation stage*. During this stage, you should take measures to ensure your best chances of preventing RLS. It is also helpful to think ahead to how you will respond to any symptoms that insist on appearing. Before your trip, it is important to consider your state of mind, time of travel, seat location, wardrobe, BOT contents, and the timing of the boarding process.

1. **State of mind:** RLS management for a long trip should begin at home. Just as you must be careful of your thoughts before going to sleep at night, you should also be aware of your thoughts before a trip.

   You may find yourself thinking, "I am dreading this long airplane trip. I will be miserable."

Try changing those thoughts to, "I can do this. I will make all the necessary trip arrangements and be sure to have a well-packed BOT. I will do my best to prevent RLS from occurring, but when it does appear, I will be ready with a reliable Plan of Attack and several good Relief Plans. By practicing *zero tolerance*, I will never spend more than a few minutes enduring RLS symptoms."

2. **Time of travel:** Whenever possible, plan to travel early in the day, when RLS attacks are less likely to occur.

3. **Aisle seats:** I prefer airlines that have reserved seating, so I can reserve an aisle seat. These airlines usually have the worst cancellation policies, but sometimes it is worth the gamble. Some airlines will make special seat accommodations for special needs travelers, such as RLSers. These changes are usually done at the boarding gate. If you cannot get an aisle seat, ask the flight attendant to find out if anyone would like to switch seats with you. I have been amazed at how willing people are to trade seats.

   If you are reserving seats for you and a travel companion, it is sometimes smart to reserve an aisle and window seat. Most people will not take the middle seat, unless there are no aisle or window seats available. If the strategy works, you will be left with more room to stretch. If someone comes for the middle seat, they are usually happy to switch it for the window seat so your companion can move next to you. Also, be aware that many of the arm rests on airplanes can be raised, giving you more room to wiggle and stretch.

4. **Exit rows and bulkhead seats:** Some RLSers like bulkhead seats, because they like to put their feet up on the wall. I would rather sit in a regular row, with room for my BOT under the seat in front of me. You can sometimes

reserve exit row seats, but usually you must remember to ask for them when you check in at the ticket counter or boarding gate. These rows almost always have more leg room. On larger airplanes, however, they often do not have a row in front of them, meaning you may not have a place for your BOT during take-off and landing.

5. **Clothing considerations:** Your travel attire can make a huge difference in your RLS experience. The rule of thumb for many travelers is to be comfortable and wear whatever will be easiest for getting through security checkpoints. Layering is always a good idea, so you are never too warm or too cold. On long airplane trips, I wear a favorite pair of thin, baggy slacks that have a comfortable elastic waist. I usually wear sandals that can be slipped off easily and I occasionally bring a pair of slippers to wear while on the airplane. Wearing loose comfortable clothing can help prevent RLS symptoms by keeping the RLSer from feeling confined or trapped.

6. **Medicines, supplements, alcohol, and caffeine:** Part of preparing for a trip is preparing your body for changes. Watch the clock and figure the appropriate moment to take medications and supplements, so they are working in your system when you need them. Pay attention to time zones and schedule your medicines so they will be effective in the new time zone, but will not leave you without treatment during your flight. Remember to consider the condition you want to be in when you reach your destination. You do not want to arrive sedated if you will be driving or need to be alert for a meeting.

   Be aware of the effects alcohol or caffeine might have on your RLS. Some people find an alcoholic drink will relax them, while others become more agitated and experience worse RLS symptoms after drinking. The same is true with caffeine. For some people, a cup of coffee will squelch RLS symptoms, while most RLSers find they need to avoid it.

7. **Fill the herbal tea mug:** If I take a morning flight, there is a good chance I will not need a mug of herbal tea. I still pack my mug and tea bags, just in case. If I sense an RLS attack coming on, I pull out the mug and ask the flight attendant to fill it with hot water. If it is an afternoon or evening flight, when RLS symptoms are most likely to occur, I have the mug filled just before I board the airplane.

    Be aware that most airport security rules do not allow you to take a mug with hot liquids through the security checkpoint. I have learned to wait and fill my tea mug after I am past the checkpoint. Also, because the hot water faucets on airplanes sometimes do not have enough clearance for a tall mug, it is best to get your hot water from a food stand or restaurant near your boarding gate.

8. **BOT management:** Make sure you have all your tricks packed and in a bag that can be easily accessed from your seat. Once you are through the security checkpoint, you can remove your BOT from your carryon so your BOT can go under the seat in front of you and your carryon can be put in the overhead compartment.

9. **Last to board:** If my seat is not reserved, I try to be in the first boarding group, so I can get an aisle seat. On some airlines, this means I need to get my boarding pass on the Internet before I leave home. If my seat is reserved, I try to be the last person to board the flight. I want to minimize the time I am sitting in my seat without the plane moving. I wait until they call the last group of people to board, and then I am the last person in that last group, even though my group was called earlier.

The only reason to rush onto an airplane where you have a reserved seat is if you want to be sure you can stow your carryon luggage in the compartment above your seat. If you are the last to board, your carryon may end up at the back of the airplane or be taken to the regular baggage compartment, out of your reach. If you choose to board early, you can claim your seat, stow your luggage, and stand in the back of the plane until all passengers are in their seats.

Plan of Attack: *Attack stage*

Following your Plan of Attack's *preparation stage*, you will start your *attack stage*. During the *attack* stage, take measures to keep yourself comfortably seated on the airplane. Some of those measures will be preventative, while others will be in response to mild RLS symptoms. When symptoms escalate, you will have to start a Relief Plan to immediately stop the symptoms. Your Plan of Attack on an airplane is critical, because it can keep you from having to resort to Relief Plans that are difficult to apply on a plane. At home, if your Plan of Attack fails, you can easily get out of bed and start a Relief Plan of walking. On an airplane, you do not always have the option to stand and go for a walk. You will need Relief Plans that work while you are seated (see the next section "Relief Plans for air travel").

As soon as you reach your seat, start the *attack stage* of your Plan of Attack. Keep yourself busy until the plane is airborne and you are allowed to get out of your seat. You could be sitting still for an hour between boarding time, waiting for clearance to take off, and then waiting for the *Fasten Seat Belt* sign to finally go off. The following tricks are some ways to keep yourself distracted while waiting for the opportunity to walk.

1. **Manage your tricks**: As soon as you are seated, inventory your BOT. Make sure your props can be reached easily. Managing your tricks will confirm your readiness to fight any RLS symptoms that insist on appearing.

2. **Eat a meal:** I find it helps to start my flight with a meal. I try to wait until we are airborne. Thinking about food keeps me distracted while I am waiting for the plane to level off. The act of eating takes up time and gets me well into the flight before I am aware of having to sit still. If we are delayed, I dig into the food before we take off.

3. **Planning:** Either at the beginning of the trip (as a distraction), or toward the end of the trip, when the *Fasten Seat Belt* sign is on and I have to sit still, I pull out maps, papers with reservation information, car rental agreements, and other trip planning material. Thinking about all my plans and figuring out what I will do when we land is a wonderful distraction.

4. **Herbal tea:** Especially on afternoon and evening flights, I have a mug of hot herbal tea. I start drinking the tea before any RLS symptoms appear. Knowing I have a constant source of something to tame my nerves is very helpful.

5. **Movies, reading, writing, and conversation:** There's nothing better than a stimulating conversation to pass the time. I have been known to ignore my BOT after starting a great conversation that continued until we pulled up to the gate at our destination. If I mention RLS, I am almost guaranteed a great conversation with the person next to me. Be careful if you try reading, writing, or watching a movie. Be sure it is something engrossing and not the type of material that aggravates your RLS. For me, leafing through the airline's shopping magazine will usually result in a major RLS attack.

6. **Beverage cart planning:** Once the *Fasten Seat Belt* sign is off, you are usually free to stand, walk, or stretch. During the beverage service, however, you may once again be trapped in your seat. The thought of becoming trapped by the cart can trigger RLS symptoms. Many times, just the sight of the beverage cart will make RLS symptoms appear. Try to time things so you are standing and stretching until the flight attendant starts servicing the row in front of yours. Sit down at the last minute, get your drink, and then feel free to stand up as soon as the cart and attendants are past your row. Even if you are not experiencing RLS symptoms when the beverage service begins, it is still wise to take the opportunity to stand and stretch before you become trapped by the cart.

Relief Plans for air travel

Relief Plans are designed to stop persistent RLS symptoms immediately. Most Relief Plans require you to stand and move around. On airplanes, you will need effective and reliable plans to stop RLS attacks without having to leave your seat.

Remember to have several Relief Plans ready to use. First use the tricks that are easiest to apply, saving more involved tricks for your later Relief Plans. Most of the following Relief Plan ideas can be used while you are seated. The last three suggestions are the only ones that involve walking.

1. **Simulate walking:** Since walking is the perfect Relief Plan trick, try using seated tricks that simulate walking. Air pillows, steppers, or the simulated action of these will help you feel as if you are walking. This trick should involve repetitions and the determination to keep your legs moving. You might want to do steadily-increasing repetitions (e.g., simulate ten steps, rest for the count of

ten, simulate twenty steps, rest for the count of ten, simulate thirty steps, rest for the count of ten, and so on). At some point, you might start at the beginning of your repetitions, but increase the speed. The goal is to keep you moving and distracted.

2. **Stretching:** Therapy bands are excellent for relieving severe RLS when you can't walk. If you stretch your leg out into the aisle, be careful to not trip anyone. Again, count the stretches and do several repetitions. Do not be afraid of calling attention to yourself. Maybe someone will ask you what you are doing and your RLS symptoms will subside while you are distracted by conversation.

3. **Snack relief:** When you use snacks as a Relief Plan, add the element of concentrating on your snacks. Try licking your sucker into a special shape. Strategically and methodically bite the limbs off your animal crackers or strip a pretzel of its last grain of salt before taking the first bite. Snack with focus, determination, and purpose. How many bites can you take of one popped kernel of corn? Remember, you are snacking for distraction, rather than sustenance. Eat peanuts one at a time, taking as many bites out of each one as possible.

4. **Sleep:** Though RLS has become known as a sleep disorder, many RLSers still say the best remedy to stop their RLS is to quickly go to sleep. When my RLS is out of control in an airplane, it is often because I am extremely tired. If I doze for a few minutes, it will usually stop the RLS symptoms. When symptoms persist, I use my neck pillow, listen to my music, and try to get a good long nap.

5. **Music:** When you use music as a Relief Plan trick, you are not just supplying background music. Remember, the idea is to focus on every sound. Bring along lyrics and try to memorize the words. Keep starting from the

beginning until you get every word correct without looking. If you dance, go over steps in your head or work out a new choreography. Thinking about leg movements can make your legs forget they are not moving. If you have seen the music video for a song, try to picture it as you listen to the music.

6. **Brushing:** Use brisk rubbing motions to snuff out urges to move. Chase the feelings, rubbing everywhere they appear with imaginary rubbing cream. Try to keep a steady brushing movement going as long as possible. The sensation of your touch and the task of keeping the motions going will distract you from the urges to move.

7. **Massage and lotion:** If brushing seems to help but you can't quite keep the motion going, try applying lotion. Rubbing in real lotion might be an easier task than chasing RLS symptoms with imaginary rubbing cream.

8. **Change your layers or shoes:** The act of putting on a sweater, taking off a jacket, or removing a sweatshirt can be sufficient distraction to stop an RLS attack. It can also help to remove your shoes or change to a pair of slippers. While you are changing shoes, be sure to give yourself a lengthy foot massage.

9. **Organize your BOT or carryon bag:** The task of organizing your BOT or carryon bag is not only distracting, but also helps you review your options for tricks. You can stay nicely distracted by balancing everything on your lap, organizing, re-packaging props, and removing trash. Make note of your next three options for Relief Plan tricks, in case you need them. While you are doing this, look for your parking garage ticket, car keys, and baggage claim tags.

During panic moments when you think, "Oh, my goodness, where are they?" your heart will race and you will get a shot of adrenaline, which might just calm your RLS symptoms.

10. **Walk:** If you can walk, do it. On long flights with in-flight movies, watch your timing. While everyone is watching the movie, it is a great time to walk. Once the movie is over, people will race to the bathroom, making standing room scarce. Another great time to walk is right after the beverage cart is put away, while everyone's tray tables are still down.

 With the current concern for airline security, some flight attendants will tell you to stay seated until a restroom is vacated or unless you have an acceptable reason to be standing. If you calmly explain your situation with RLS, they will usually accommodate your need to stand. You might be asked to stand at your seat, in the galley, or somewhere out of the way, but you will usually be allowed to remain out of your seat, as long as the *Fasten Seat Belt* sign remains off.

11. **Pit stops:** A trip to the bathroom can provide many distractions. Take your time. Wash your hands and face, comb your hair, brush your teeth, or apply makeup. The object is to stay busy and distracted. Do anything that will help you stop thinking about sitting still. Unless you are a petite person, you will be nicely distracted with the task of turning, sitting, and using your arms (without bruising your elbows) in a confined space.

12. **Conversations in the galley:** I have relieved many persistent RLS attacks by standing in the galley and explaining RLS to flight attendants and other passengers. If you can share some printed RLS information (which you just happen to have with you), you might gain a little credibility and earn more standing time. Maybe a future RLS traveler will benefit from your efforts to educate the crew.

Pay attention to the return trip

During an outbound flight, many RLSers find it easy to manage symptoms. At the start of a trip, our adrenaline and excitement levels are high. Distracted by new sights and sounds, we are full of thoughts about where we are going and what we will be doing. Our outbound trips are often scheduled early in the day (when RLS symptoms are least likely), in an attempt to allow time to complete business or start enjoying ourselves early. In anticipation of the long trip, we tend to be careful to avoid RLS aggravators and to have all of our best tricks ready to use.

After a good outbound trip experience, RLSers often get a false sense of security. We figure that if there were no RLS symptoms on the way out, there won't be any on the way home. Consequently, we are usually not as prepared to prevent or respond to RLS attacks on the return trip.

As we approach our return trip, many variables contribute to aggravated RLS symptoms. We tend to travel late in the day so we can finish business or take advantage of every minute of our vacation. Our normal routines are usually disrupted after sleeping in new surroundings, eating new foods, and keeping different schedules. Add to this the fact that we might be overly confident after our success on the outbound trip. Often, it is during the last leg of the journey (e.g., the puddle-jumper, taxi, train, car ride home) that we experience the worst RLS symptoms of the entire trip.

RLS symptoms started during a return trip can continue through the first night you are home. Though you look forward to the comfort of your bed and expect to finally sleep soundly, you might be surprised to find a raging case of RLS still plaguing you. The trip is not over until you have slept one night at home, so be ready with a plan.

Another typical problem on a return trip is that your mind is tired and vulnerable to the *RLS bully*'s urges to move. Your desire might be to rest and not think of anything until you get home, but you might be better off planning some mental distractions or going to sleep as quickly as possible.

Some people will start thinking of what they will do when they get home. This can also become an RLS aggravator. Being trapped on the airplane, anticipating upcoming deadlines and chores, can set off a wild RLS attack. Plan for these last moments of your trip, deciding how you can stay calm and avoid becoming restless.

With careful planning and a well developed approach to using your BOT, you will be able to prevent many RLS attacks and manage those that are persistent. Be diligent about planning your return trip strategies. The RLSers who contacted me and helped me develop these travel suggestions, found their planning paid off with a more enjoyable experience than they had anticipated. When you get back from your trip, drop me a line (jill@rlsrebel.com) and let me know how you did. Perhaps you will discover new tricks we can pass along to other RLS travelers. Bon voyage!

To Those Who Support Us

I THOUGHT I HAD a great idea when I asked my husband to write this chapter as a peer support chapter, from one Restless Legs Syndrome (RLS) supporter to another. He's a smart man. He told me to do it myself. Being a smart woman, however, and knowing how well my husband has supported me during the last thirty years of dealing with my RLS idiosyncrasies, I twisted his arm one more time.

He still refused to write the chapter, but he answered my main question: "If you were going to give advice to RLS supporters, what would you tell them?"

Figuring I had managed my RLS well and had been easy to support over the years, I expected a short list of suggestions. So much for that thought! Here is his advice to those of you who support RLSers (people who experience RLS symptoms). For the rest of this chapter, I will be using the pronoun *her* to refer to the RLSer. My husband started it (in his comments below), and I am just following his lead—for once.

1. Do not be surprised if you find yourself wanting to scream, "Sit still!"

2. Let her drive whenever she wants.

3. Give the aisle seat to her. Even if your legs are longer, you will be happier if you don't have to keep letting her out to walk.

4. Don't be offended if she won't let you touch her when she's trying to get to sleep.

5. Don't be surprised when your RLSer leaves your bed during the night and seems happier to be awake, playing computer games, doing chores, or soaking in a bath.

6. Don't expect routine bedtimes, but encourage them.

7. Don't be hurt if she resists going to bed with you. It's not you she's avoiding.

8. Accept the fact she has less energy than others. She would love to be energetic and lively, if she could only get a decent night's sleep.

9. Don't be surprised if she shows little enthusiasm for a long drive in the country, a flight to Australia, or cuddling in front of the TV.

10. Expect her to be frustrated and short-tempered, due to sleep deprivation or depression.

11. Learn about RLS so you will understand things like her tendency to sleep best from 4:00 until 9:00 A.M.

12. Realize she may not be great company on a car trip. When she is not driving, she may be sleeping, busily involved in distractive tricks, or periodically yelling, "Stop this car! Now!"

13. Get used to sharing space with her Bag of Tricks (BOT).

14. If she gets into bed and starts breathing deeply, don't get excited. It may be part of her Plan of Attack for going to sleep.

15. Don't be surprised when she shrinks back and vehemently refuses the chocolate candy and red wine you bought for a romantic night. She may have learned chocolates and red wine can trigger her RLS attacks.

16. If she says she's too frustrated for sex, tell her you read somewhere that it's a great distraction trick for RLS.

17. When she mentions *the RLS beast* or *the RLS bully*, don't expect to see another person.

18. If she is using medications for RLS, be prepared to interpret side effects from the medications.

19. Don't be surprised if her usual RLS relief tricks suddenly stop working.

20. If you are still single and thinking of marrying an RLSer, think again. It runs in families. Your children may be poor sleepers and your grandbabies may scream all night. It happened to us, and it can happen to you, too. Worse yet, she could end up writing a book about RLS, and you will only know her from the back of her head as she spends hour after hour at the computer.

I'm sorry about number 20. When we got to that point, we were having a good laugh about how ridiculous this situation can become. Do not hesitate to marry an RLSer. Just know what you are getting into and be prepared. I have to say, the list amazed me. I forgot how much my husband understands about RLS and how long he has been at my side, supporting me in my RLS survival. He could have written this book—and it would have been much shorter. As usual, I have more to add to the subject.

Prepare for the role of RLS rebel supporter

There is a difference between knowing an RLSer and deciding to support an RLSer. Many people unexpectedly find themselves in an RLS support role. They may know nothing about the syndrome or have any ideas about how to bring relief or comfort to their RLSer. Whether you are new to the job or looking for ways to improve support efforts you have given for years, I suggest you look at it as if you were starting a new job.

Along with a good job description, you will need to know a great deal about the business (RLS), the unique problems of the company (your RLSer's symptoms), the program and goals (treatments), and the working relationship you will have with the management (your RLSer). Learn what you can offer the position, what the position will require of you, and what makes this position unique. The following tips are ways you can approach your role of RLS supporter with the seriousness and determination you might put into a new job.

1. Prepare for the job by reading the rest of this book and researching other books and websites about Restless Legs Syndrome.

2. Learn the lingo of the job (e.g., Bag of Tricks Approach [BOTA], tricks, beast of RLS, RLS bully, Reduction Plan, RLS notebook).

3. Learn about your RLSer's symptoms and treatments, just as you would learn about the unique problems and solutions at a new job.

4. Learn about job relationships. Who is in charge (you or your RLSer)? Who are your peers (are there doctors, support groups, or others who are also supporting your RLSer)?

5. Ask for a job description. Learn what your role will be and how you are expected to deliver your support.

6. Learn the ropes before suggesting too many changes to the program. The RLSer may have years of personal experience and valuable insights.

7. Respect the management (your RLSer) and the company (RLS). Recognize the challenge you will face, dealing

with such a "shifty" syndrome (I know, bad pun). Avoid viewing your RLSer as a helpless victim to be rescued. You are there to help, not to take over the company.

8. Ask about your pay. If you get a good answer, please do not mention it to my husband. He is still pestering me about his fringe benefits.

The many hats you wear

Decisions about your job description should be based on communication and understanding between you and your RLSer. Some of us are good at being personal caregivers, while others are more inclined to provide information or technical resources. As you review ways to fit into the program and provide valuable support, consider the many types of support roles you could fill.

1. **Researcher:** Your RLSer might appreciate your efforts to research and organize RLS information. You can listen to the questions and search for answers, saving your RLSer time and energy.

2. **Coach:** Sometimes people need coaches to help them stick to their programs and continue developing skills. Be sure, however, to coach your RLSer in the program of her choice. It would not make sense to coach an athlete in high jumping if she wanted to do pole vaulting. By the same token, you would not want to coach an RLSer to primarily use prescription medications if she wanted to focus on using alternatives, or vice versa.

3. **Cheerleader:** It may seem silly, but sometimes the support we need most is a good *atta girl*. When you are tired of trying and you're thinking of giving up, a little encouragement goes a long way.

4. **Mental focus partner:** One of the best RLS tricks is to concentrate on something that keeps the RLSer's mind

too busy to be bothered by ridiculous urges to move. It takes practice and determination to develop the skill of concentration, but it's one that can be used in many other situations (e.g., I used it to prevent anxiety when I woke up from surgery and later, when I had allergic reactions from chemotherapy and thought I would go crazy from the horrible itching). It may be beneficial to you and your RLSer to work together in developing the skill of concentration.

5. **Damage control expert:** Due to exhaustion, effects from medications, depression, or severe RLS attacks, RLSers sometimes feel as if they are on a sinking ship. You may be most supportive by helping your RLSer see what's going well and pointing out variables that can be adjusted to bring relief (e.g., remind her she was given Benadryl while she was ill, gently point out the chocolate she ate).

6. **Official reminder:** You can help your RLSer remember to approach any RLS-provoking situation with a BOTA.

7. **Record keeper:** Ask your RLSer if she would like you to contribute to her RLS notebook or take charge of keeping the notebook up to date.

Use the RLS Rebel Program

It will help your support efforts if you become familiar with the RLS Rebel Program. The program follows an outline that guides the RLSer in managing variables and strategies. The RLSer is encouraged to keep a file system or notebook, using each part of the program outline as a file or a section of her RLS rebel notebook.

The following suggestions are ways an RLS supporter can implement the RLS Rebel Program Outline. Remember, the extent to which you do any of these supportive tasks depends on the extent to which your RLSer *wants* you involved in her program. Offer to help, but do not impose.

The REDUCTION PLAN

Step 1: Reduce PANIC *(Get educated)*
Be a part of the learning, researching, and recording process. Collect articles and keep a list of topics to research. If you attend doctor appointments, offer to take notes. Remind your RLSer to make a list of questions to be answered at the next doctor's appointment or to be added to the list of research topics.

Step 2: Reduce CHAOS *(Analyze symptoms)*
Sometimes the supporter can see things the RLSer can't. You may be able to help analyze, describe, and predict RLS attacks so better treatments and responses can be planned.

Step 3: Reduce SYMPTOMS *(Identify coexisting ailments)*
Encourage your RLSer to have a good physical to identify coexisting ailments that may be aggravating RLS symptoms. Note which symptoms belong to which ailments and which symptoms should be relieved by each treatment. Offer to help chart symptoms, ailments, and treatments.

Step 4: Reduce DEFICIENCIES *(Adjust supplements)*
You may be able to help a great deal by doing research on supplements and recording what supplements and combinations have been tried. It's also helpful to maintain a list of things to try in the future.

Step 5: Reduce AGGRAVATORS *(Identify triggers)*
Help your RLSer identify and avoid aggravators (e.g., irritating foods, medicines, people, chairs, environments, clothes, reading material, certain types of movies or TV shows).

Step 6: Reduce SITUATIONS *(Prioritize needs)*
Help your RLSer identify activities that are often interrupted by RLS symptoms. Together, you can prioritize and target important situations to treat. You can support your RLSer in efforts to avoid certain situations until she has better control over her RLS.

The BAG OF TRICKS APPROACH (BOTA)

Step 1: GATHER YOUR TRICKS *(List all treatment options)* Familiarize yourself with RLS tricks, including pharmaceutical or non-pharmaceutical therapies. Help your RLSer maintain lists of prop tricks and no-prop tricks.

Step 2: PACK YOUR BAGS *(Match treatments with activities)* If your RLSer is using prescription medications, help her remember to match the treatment with the desired effects. Make sure she isn't taking a sleeping pill to relieve RLS symptoms and then expecting to stay awake during a concert. Before beginning an RLS-provoking activity, help your RLSer remember to gather the tricks that are most helpful during that activity.

Step 3: PLAN OF ATTACK *(Your plan for getting through an activity)* Familiarize yourself with your RLSer's BOTA and coach her through the process. Help her prepare for at-rest activities so she has the greatest chance of preventing RLS symptoms. Then encourage her to start her tricks early so she has the best chance of getting through the at-rest act activity.

Step 4: RELIEF PLANS *(Your plan to stop symptoms, immediately)* If your RLSer's Plan of Attack fails and RLS symptoms escalate, she has to quickly apply reliable Relief Plan tricks. Ask if there is anything you can do to help, but don't be surprised if your RLSer exclaims, "I just have to move!" If you are driving and can pull the car over safely, let your RLSer get out and stretch. If you are watching a movie at home and can pause the DVD, your RLSer will appreciate the chance to move around, stop the RLS symptoms and not miss any of the movie. In fact, if you detect RLS symptoms starting, you might suggest some of these solutions before the symptoms have a chance to escalate.

When my husband stops a movie and says, "I need a break," I'm always grateful. I hate to always be the one needing the break.

Sometimes you have to take charge

If your RLSer is bedridden, you may have to assume greater responsibility for preventing, detecting, and responding to RLS symptoms. Your RLSer may be tired, ill, or incapacitated, but still experiencing severe RLS symptoms and in desperate need of relief. It will help a great deal if you understand the concepts of the RLS Rebel Program (e.g., *zero tolerance, bully noise*) and can use them effectively to provide your RLSer symptom relief. As soon as you see your bedridden RLSer wiggling uncomfortably from RLS, you can try distracting her, massaging her legs, or helping her stand or stretch. It will also help if you know what variables aggravate RLS and make sure those variables are adjusted or avoided.

It may become your responsibility to help the RLSer wiggle or become distracted, in order to quickly stop the urges. If your RLSer can get out of bed and walk, be aware of possible side effects from medications and illness. Her lack of stability may make walking a less desirable RLS trick.

If walking isn't an option, a special BOT will be needed. For more information on what can be done in situations where RLSers are bedridden, see the earlier chapter, "Special Situations."

Socialization and emotional health

RLSers often make unconscious adjustments to accommodate their RLS symptoms. After many attempts to go to the movies with friends, enjoy the opera, travel, or take part in meetings, dinners, or lectures, an RLSer may begin declining invitations and refusing to plan future activities. In the worst-case scenario, the person may become depressed and suicidal.

As the supporter of an RLSer, you may be able to encourage open communication regarding changes you have observed in her social involvement and emotional health. It's possible there are simple adjustments that will make things better, once you both realize the problem. I began resisting long car trips until my husband realized how uncomfortable they were for me. Once he said, "You can drive anytime you want," I was much more excited about future trips.

For years, I allowed my husband to take the aisle seat at a theater or the end seat in a restaurant booth because his legs were longer. At the time, I did not realize I could have been taking steps to prevent *my leg thing* from bothering me. I never imagined he could be comfortable with his legs still and no way to stretch or get out of his seat. Instead, I got to where I disliked going to movies and restaurants. These days, I take seats that allow me movement and freedom to stand when I need to stretch and distract myself.

If communication and adjustments are not enough, and your RLSer continues to withdraw, it may be a good idea to seek help from a health professional.

Supporting children who have RLS

If you are a teacher, parent, or friend of a child with RLS, read the earlier chapter on helping children deal with RLS. Just as adults can withdraw rather than communicate and figure out simple adjustments, children can seem to have behavior problems and do things that do not appear to make sense. A reluctance to go on a field trip or sleep at a friend's house could be due to frustration with RLS symptoms. What seems to be an attention deficit disorder or behavioral problem could be a persistent case of irresistible RLS urges to wiggle. Rowdy behavior on a driving trip could be a sign of an RLS attack, rather than a devilish urge to get siblings into trouble. You can support a child with RLS by helping the child learn about the syndrome and how to become an RLS rebel with a full BOT.

Relationships

As with any difficult ailment or trauma, RLS can seriously threaten relationships. It is not unusual for couples to complain their relationship has been ruined because they can't share the same bed. Talking about it may help, but when you live with an RLSer, your communication can be affected by frustration, sleep deprivation, depression, or panic. Do not take this personally. Try to find ways to diffuse tension and distract your RLSer while you communicate. Going for a walk with your RLSer is a great way to distract and talk at the same time. If communication is not possible, seek counseling.

If you and your RLSer are on different sleeping schedules or using separate bedrooms, it may help you both get sleep, but it will take a greater effort to keep communication open. Many RLSers spend hours being alone at night, walking the floors, or sitting at the computer. In the morning, it's not unusual for the RLSer to finally sleep, while the partner gets up at a relatively normal time. Before long, if the couple is not careful, it is easy to miss valuable moments when conversations could have taken place. Insist on making time to talk.

Never assume your RLSer's absence from bed is a reflection of her desire to be with you. Most of us would love to stay in bed all night, sleeping peacefully, if only we could. Your RLSer may be staying awake and avoiding your bed because she does not want her wiggling to wake you. Make sure you talk about feelings and intentions so there is no misunderstanding.

Appearances can be deceiving

Do not assume your RLSer is free of RLS symptoms just because she sleeps at night or sits through a movie. She may be employing a full BOT and making many adjustments in order to appear normal. RLSers don't get over RLS—they just get better at fighting back and surviving.

One night, after a long day at a Restless Legs Syndrome Foundation national conference, I was sitting in the hot tub with several other conference goers. One of them was a beautiful lady who had severe RLS, along with what seemed like an endless number of other ailments.

Intending to give her a compliment, I said, "You look great, considering all the things that are wrong with you."

She looked as if I had just stuck a dagger in her heart and said, "Jill! I would have thought *you*, of all people, would understand that our pain and suffering does not have to show on the outside in order for us to be hurting inside."

I did not mean to suggest she was not hurting or suffering, but that she looked better than I would have looked if I had to deal with all her ailments.

That night, I learned a lesson about how easy it is to have preconceived notions about what a person should look like when suffering from frustrating ailments. A sleep deprived, frustrated RLSer does not necessarily look awful. When a person is trying hard to survive, a little attention to makeup, hairdo, wardrobe, and keeping a positive, determined attitude can make that person appear to be better off than she really is.

Just be a friend

I want to thank you for all your efforts to support your RLSer. This crazy syndrome is hard enough to understand when experienced firsthand. I can only imagine what it's like for you, trying to support someone with RLS. I hope the suggestions in this chapter will support *your* efforts. When all is said and done, there is one suggestion that shines above all the rest. You probably already have this one down pat, but I want to share a story as a way of stressing how much your friendship and support can mean to an RLSer.

Many years ago, when my children were preschoolers, I was active in facilitating two parenting groups. One group dealt with child abuse issues and the other was a group for mothers who were breastfeeding their babies. I was fortunate to be able to represent the child abuse group at the National Conference on Child Abuse and Neglect.

I had several ideas of what I wanted to learn at the conference, but I figured if I came away from the conference with one good bit of information, it would have been worth my trip. The most important thing I wanted to find was some information to help one of the mothers in the nursing mother's group. She had a child who refused to eat and the child had stopped growing.

I was thrilled when I discovered an exhibit with a huge sign saying, "Failure to Thrive Syndrome." Finally, I would be able to take home pertinent information to help that mother and her baby. I rushed up to the table and explained my situation to two ladies manning the exhibit. I begged them to give me pamphlets, videos, or whatever material they had on the syndrome. It was the mid-1980s, so I could not go home and search the Internet for information.

When I asked, "What can I do for this mother?" their answer was, "Go home and be her friend."

I protested, explaining I was a group leader and I needed to give this mother advice, answers, or information.

They repeated, "Go home and be her friend."

Again, I protested, "There must be something I can tell her to mention to her doctor. A test? A drug? A therapy?"

A third time, I heard, "Go home and be her friend."

Frustrated and furious, I left the exhibit. When I got home, I visited the mother and baby. I explained how close I had come to finding answers and how furious I had been at the ridiculous exhibit ladies who refused to share their knowledge and secrets.

I was shocked when the mother looked at me and said, "Jill, they were right."

As it turns out, she knew her child's problem was called Failure to Thrive Syndrome. Her doctors had done all the tests. She and her husband were already doing everything in their power.

She explained it to me, saying, "What I really need is for you and the other mothers to believe in me. I need you to believe that I am not crazy and I am not a bad mother. My baby's growth problems and lack of eating are not my fault. What I need right now, more than anything, is a friend."

In years to come, that lady gave birth to two more sons, both of whom grew into handsome, strong, healthy, good-sized young men. Her first son became an active and treasured member of the family, but he never grew and thrived like the others. Evidently, his mother had the answers and knew what she had to do. She just needed the support of a friend.

What does this have to do with supporting your RLSer? Whether you become totally involved in your RLSer's rebel program or you support her quietly from the sideline, the most important thing you can do is to *just be a friend*. Understand. Listen. Believe in your RLSer and her fight for control. She is not crazy. She just lives with a crazy syndrome. If you do no more than just be her friend, you will be giving her the most important support of all.

Parting Thoughts

I LIVED WITH MY *leg thing* (aka *my growing pains)* for forty-six years before learning what it was. In 1998, when I first learned about Restless Legs Syndrome (RLS), reports claimed RLS symptoms occurred mostly in middle-aged people. There was little recognition of childhood RLS or of the tendency for RLS to be experienced by many within the same family. During the next eight years, research and feedback (from RLSers, their families, and healthcare providers) added volumes to what we knew about RLS. There are times when I think RLS information is developing at a snail's pace, but there are times when I am thrilled with major changes in thinking, awareness, knowledge, and treatments for RLS.

People used to argue about how we needed to change the name from RLS to something that sounded more serious, just so doctors would not laugh at us when we told them we thought we had Restless Legs Syndrome. Today, very few people are laughing about it. Research is continuing and new discoveries are being made all over the world. I do not know if we will find solutions in my lifetime, but we have already improved our quality of life and our hope for the future beyond my imagination.

Help find the cure

Your feedback to RLS doctors and researchers is extremely helpful. Since so little about RLS can be clinically tested, a good deal of their information comes from observations made by RLSers and their families. As an example, they no longer say RLS is only a problem in midlife. They no longer say prescription medications are the only treatment for severe RLS. They recognize a person can have mild RLS, but suddenly have severe episodes when traveling or having surgery. These changes in thinking did not develop in a test tube, but came from feedback RLSers provided through the years.

Along with providing good feedback to healthcare providers and researchers, you can help by volunteering to run a local RLS support group. Contact the Restless Legs Syndrome Foundation and they will help you in your efforts to support others. Help your doctor, local hospital, or nursing home by providing information and offering support to other RLSers and their healthcare providers. Observations and feedback you gather from your support group efforts may help further RLS information and lead us closer to a cure.

Consider taking part in a study or research project. From time to time, researchers are looking for participants in studies for new medications, new diagnostic information, and quality of life surveys. The RLS Foundation can direct you to studies that need participants.

Consider donating your brain to RLS research. Many RLSers have made arrangements to have their brains studied by RLS researchers. Donated brains have already led to information (e.g., differences in content of iron in brains of RLSers and non-RLSers) that may significantly change future treatments. Contact the RLS Foundation for information on brain banks and donation programs.

And finally, you can help find a cure by giving financial support. As a start, consider joining the RLS Foundation. Your yearly membership fee will support research and educational programs, while keeping you informed of new discoveries, via *Nightwalkers*, the foundation's quarterly newsletter.

Become a more skillful RLS rebel

When I first discovered the name *RLS* and began my conscious fight against it, my RLS symptoms had become unbearable. Sleep deprivation had become a major problem and my health was suffering. Today, I still have RLS attacks, but the RLS Rebel Program helps me stay in control of my experiences with RLS. There is hope that we can improve our coping skills faster than our RLS symptoms will worsen.

Be still!

Many of the concepts in this book suggest we keep our minds and bodies busy. We know that if we just relax or be still, we are more likely to experience an RLS attack. An empty mind is a mind that will be filled with the ridiculous and obnoxious taunts of the *RLS bully*.

Despite this knowledge, my ultimate rebel goal is to retrain myself to sit still and stay put.

I am not sure this is possible, but I know there are times I can say to myself, "Hey, stop it! You are not going anywhere. Just settle down, behave, and be still!"

I am working on discouraging my fight-or-flight response and encouraging my ability to be still.

I keep telling myself, "It's okay to just *be*, with no place to go and nothing to do."

And yet, even as I type this, I feel the RLS feelings telling me, "Run!"

RLS affirmations and reminders

RLS itself is not fatal.

I have to believe my tricks will work.

RLS is not welcome in my body!

Zero tolerance is my first and best defense.

RLS is an obnoxious bully I shall control!

The more I know, the more empowered I will be.

I am not a helpless victim!

Though exhausted, I am an empowered RLS rebel.

Best wishes for restful moments and peaceful nights

If you are struggling with your RLS Rebel Program and want support, feel free to email me (jill@rlsrebel.com) or contact me through my website: http://rlsrebel.com.

I love hearing what others have learned and I continue to learn by helping others. I truly hope this survival guide and the RLS Rebel Program will be needless in the near future. I pray a cause and cure will be discovered, and the treatment will be easy.

Best wishes to you—for quality sleep, restful moments, and peaceful nights.

Printed in the United States
101532LV00005B/75/A